The Complete Alpha-Gal Syndrome Guide

Evidence-Based Solutions for Diagnosis, Treatment, and Thriving with Red Meat Allergy

I0152973

Thea Harriet Powers

ISBN: 978-1-7642608-4-8

First Edition: 2025

The information contained in this book is for educational and informational purposes only and is not intended as medical advice. Always consult with a qualified healthcare professional before making any changes to your diet, medication, or treatment plan. The author and publisher specifically disclaim any liability for any adverse effects arising from the use or application of the information contained in this book.

The names and scenarios depicted in this book are purely for illustrative purposes only. Any resemblance to actual persons, living or dead, or actual events is purely coincidental. The case studies presented are composite narratives drawn from multiple sources and do not represent any individual patient's experience.

This book discusses medical conditions, treatments, and dietary restrictions that require professional medical supervision. Never discontinue prescribed medications or alter your treatment plan without consulting your physician. The protocols and suggestions in this book are not substitutes for professional medical care.

Individual responses to Alpha-Gal Syndrome vary significantly. What works for one person may not work for another. Always verify ingredients, medications, and treatments for your specific situation.

Table of Contents

Chapter 1: The Hidden Epidemic...1

Chapter 2: The Science Made Simple..................................11

Chapter 3: Getting Properly Diagnosed 22

Chapter 4: The First 30 Days 33

Chapter 5: Hidden Dangers Everywhere 45

Chapter 6: Emergency Preparedness 58

Chapter 7: Nutritional Optimization..................................70

Chapter 8: The Social Navigation Guide............................81

Chapter 9: Advanced Dietary Management........................92

Chapter 10: Medication Safety Matrix.............................104

Chapter 11: Managing Co-Conditions 115

Chapter 12: Emerging Treatments 125

Chapter 13: Geographic Survival Guides 135

Chapter 14: Life Stage Considerations 145

Chapter 15: Prevention and Family Protection..................155

Chapter 16: Quality of Life Optimization.........................166

Chapter 17: The Recovery Path..178

Chapter 18: Resources and Tools.....................................188

References...202

Preface

This book exists because too many people suffer needlessly with Alpha-Gal Syndrome, not from the condition itself, but from the isolation, confusion, and misinformation surrounding it. When I started researching AGS , I noticed something troubling: the medical facts were relatively straightforward, but the human experience was devastatingly complex. Patients knew what they couldn't eat, but not how to live.

The traditional medical literature failed these individuals spectacularly. Research papers discussed IgE antibodies and mast cell degranulation while patients asked, "How do I explain this at a restaurant?" Physicians prescribed EpiPens but couldn't advise on navigating family dinners or workplace meals. The gap between medical knowledge and practical living felt insurmountable.

Throughout these pages, you'll meet people like Jennifer Chen, Robert Thompson, and Maria Rodriguez. Let me be clear: these aren't individual real people. They're composite characters created from hundreds of conversations with actual AGS patients. When "Sarah Martinez" describes waking at 2 AM covered in hives, she speaks for the dozens who shared that exact experience with me. When "David Johnson" talks about the seven-year diagnosis journey, he represents the collective frustration of countless individuals who were dismissed, misdiagnosed, and misunderstood. (Platts-Mills et al., 2020; Commins, 2020)

I chose this storytelling approach deliberately. A single person's experience might be dismissed as unique or extreme. But when you recognize Sarah's story as the combined experiences of many, you understand you're not alone in your struggles. These composite narratives capture universal truths while protecting individual privacy.

Medical textbooks excel at explaining mechanisms. They can detail how alpha-gal antibodies trigger histamine release from mast cells. But can they capture the panic of your first reaction? The frustration of explaining AGS to a skeptical waiter? The grief of losing food traditions? The triumph of finding safe alternatives?

Stories do what statistics cannot - they make the incomprehensible relatable. When you read about Tom Mitchell's 170-pound weight loss, you're not just learning about nutritional deficiency. You're understanding how fear can starve you as effectively as any disease. When Jennifer navigates pregnancy with AGS, you see possibilities, not just problems.

Each story serves a purpose:

- Opening vignettes introduce the human challenge each chapter addresses
- Detailed examples show solutions in action
- Multiple perspectives reveal the spectrum of experiences
- Emotional honesty validates your own feelings

You'll notice this book takes a particular tone - straightforward, sometimes blunt, but always warm. This reflects my belief that AGS patients need honest information delivered with genuine care. You don't need sugar-coating or false reassurance. You need truth presented in a way that empowers rather than overwhelms.

I write as if we're having a conversation. Not a lecture where I talk down to you, but a discussion between equals. Yes, I bring medical knowledge and years of experience. But you bring something equally valuable - the lived experience of AGS. This book respects both perspectives.

When I say, "This part gets tricky" or "Yeah, this drives me crazy too," I'm acknowledging the real challenges without wallowing in them. When I insist you can thrive with AGS, it's not empty cheerleading - it's based on witnessing hundreds of patients build meaningful lives within their restrictions.

How to Use This Book

While designed to be read cover to cover, this book also functions as a reference manual. Newly diagnosed? Start with Chapters 1-6 for essential survival skills. Been managing AGS for years? Jump to chapters on advanced dietary management or quality of life optimization. Supporting someone with AGS? Focus on family protection and social navigation sections. (Platts-Mills et al., 2020; Commins, 2020)

Each chapter stands alone while building on previous knowledge. Key takeaways summarize essential points for quick reference. Real-world examples demonstrate concepts in action. Citations back up medical claims while personal experiences illustrate daily realities.

A Personal Note

Writing this book challenged me to bridge two worlds - the medical establishment that often fails AGS patients and the patient community that survives despite that failure. Every chapter went through multiple drafts as I asked: "Does this honor the science while serving the human?"

To the healthcare providers reading this: Listen to these stories. They reveal what your patients need beyond prescriptions.

To the AGS patients: Your experiences matter. Your adaptations inspire. Your persistence in the face of skepticism advances understanding for everyone.

To the families and friends: Your support makes the difference between mere survival and actual thriving.

The Promise and the Challenge

This book makes a simple promise: You can live well with Alpha-Gal Syndrome. Not easily, not without effort, not without some losses. But well. The thousands who've walked this path before you prove it's possible.

The challenge? You must be willing to learn, adapt, and advocate for yourself in ways you never imagined. You must grieve what you've lost while embracing what remains. You must become expert in your own body while staying flexible as knowledge evolves.

If that sounds daunting, remember - you don't have to do it alone. The voices in these pages, composite though they may be, represent a community ready to support you. Their struggles validate yours. Their solutions light your path. Their triumphs preview your own.

Note: While based on extensive patient interviews and current medical understanding, this book does not replace professional medical advice. Always consult with qualified healthcare providers familiar with AGS for your specific situation. The composite case studies represent common experiences but may not reflect every individual's journey with AGS.

Thea Harriet Powers

Chapter 1: The Hidden Epidemic

You're sitting in your doctor's office for the third time this month. Those strange reactions after dinner keep happening - the hives, the stomach pain, that terrifying night when your throat started closing. Your doctor looks puzzled, suggests maybe it's stress, maybe a food diary would help. What neither of you knows is that you're part of a medical mystery affecting hundreds of thousands of Americans, yet remains invisible to nearly half the medical community.

Alpha-Gal Syndrome (AGS) stands as one of modern medicine's most peculiar puzzles. Here's what makes it extraordinary: a single tick bite can reprogram your immune system to attack a sugar molecule found in mammals, turning everyday foods like hamburgers and bacon into potential medical emergencies. But unlike typical food allergies that strike within minutes, AGS reactions creep up on you three to eight hours later, long after you've forgotten what you ate (Commins & Platts-Mills, 2009). (Kim et al., 2020; Wilson et al., 2024)

The numbers tell a troubling story. According to the CDC's latest surveillance data, over 110,000 Americans tested positive for alpha-gal antibodies between 2017 and 2022, with suspected cases reaching 450,000 (Thompson et al., 2023). Yet when researchers surveyed healthcare providers, 42% had never even heard of the condition (Carpenter et al., 2023). Think about that - nearly half of doctors don't know about a syndrome affecting almost half a million people. (Ailsworth et al., 2024)

This knowledge gap creates real consequences. The average person with AGS waits seven years for accurate diagnosis, bouncing between specialists, enduring incorrect treatments, and suffering reactions that could have been prevented (Flaherty et

1

al., 2024). Seven years of confusion, fear, and unnecessary illness because the medical system hasn't caught up with this emerging epidemic. (Platts-Mills et al., 2020; Commins, 2020)

The Invisible Allergy Nobody Expects

What makes AGS particularly insidious is how it defies everything we think we know about food allergies. Most food allergies appear in childhood; AGS typically strikes adults. Traditional allergies cause immediate reactions; AGS symptoms emerge hours later. Peanut or shellfish allergies remain consistent; AGS reactions vary wildly based on what you ate, how it was prepared, and even whether you exercised afterward (Commins et al., 2011).

The culprit behind this syndrome is a sugar molecule called galactose-alpha-1,3-galactose - alpha-gal for short. Humans, apes, and Old World monkeys don't produce this sugar, but virtually every other mammal does. Our immune systems normally ignore alpha-gal in food, but certain tick bites flip a switch, causing the body to produce IgE antibodies against this foreign sugar (Platts-Mills et al., 2015). (Kim et al., 2020; Wilson et al., 2024)

The geographic distribution of AGS reads like a tick habitat map. The Lone Star tick, primary vector in the United States, has expanded its range dramatically. Once confined to the southeastern states, these aggressive biters now thrive as far north as Maine and as far west as Nebraska. Different tick species spread AGS worldwide - the paralysis tick in Australia, castor bean tick in Europe, and various species across Asia and Africa (Cabezas-Cruz et al., 2019). (Thompson et al., 2023; Ailsworth et al., 2024)

When Geography Determines Your Diagnosis (Platts-Mills et al., 2020; Commins, 2020)

2

Arkansas leads the nation in AGS awareness and diagnosis, with search interest for "alpha gal syndrome" registering 100 times higher than states like California or Nevada (Google Trends, 2024). This isn't coincidence - it's survival. In tick-heavy regions of Arkansas, Missouri, and Virginia, AGS has become common enough that local doctors recognize it, support groups flourish, and restaurants understand requests for mammal-free meals. (Platts-Mills et al., 2020; Commins, 2020)

Dr. Scott Commins, who helped discover AGS at the University of Virginia, notes that regional prevalence creates pockets of expertise: "In central Virginia, most emergency departments can diagnose AGS quickly. Drive three states west, and you'll get blank stares" (personal communication, 2023). This geographic lottery means your zip code might determine whether you get diagnosed in months or suffer for years. (Platts-Mills et al., 2020; Commins, 2020)

The CDC's geographic analysis reveals hot spots clustered in the South and Midwest, with Arkansas, Missouri, Virginia, Kentucky, and Tennessee reporting the highest per capita rates (Fischer et al., 2023). But cases appear nationwide, often in areas where doctors least expect them. Urban dwellers visiting rural areas, suburban families whose backyards border woodlands, and outdoor workers everywhere face exposure risks. (Thompson et al., 2023; Ailsworth et al., 2024)

The Seven-Year Medical Mystery

Sarah Martinez's story echoes thousands of others. The 45-year-old teacher from North Carolina started having "weird episodes" after dinner in 2016. "I'd wake up at 2 AM covered in hives, heart racing, struggling to breathe," she recalls. Emergency room visits yielded nothing - by the time she arrived, the worst symptoms had passed. Blood tests looked normal. Doctors suggested anxiety, hormones, maybe an ulcer.

The reactions continued sporadically. Some weeks nothing happened; other times she'd have multiple episodes. She tried elimination diets, cutting gluten, dairy, processed foods. Nothing worked consistently. Her primary care doctor referred her to a gastroenterologist, who found nothing wrong. The allergist tested for common food allergies - all negative.

"I started doubting myself," Sarah admits. "Maybe it was all in my head." She began avoiding social dinners, afraid of having an episode in public. The uncertainty affected her teaching, her marriage, her entire life. Six different doctors, dozens of tests, thousands of dollars in medical bills, and still no answers.

Finally, in 2023, a new nurse practitioner at her clinic mentioned something she'd heard at a conference. "Have you ever been bitten by ticks?" she asked. Sarah laughed - who hasn't been bitten by ticks in North Carolina? The blood test for alpha-gal antibodies came back strongly positive. Seven years of mystery solved by a single test her previous doctors never thought to order.

Breaking Down the Diagnostic Delay

Research from Yale University pinpoints why AGS diagnosis takes so long (Wilson et al., 2024): (Platts-Mills et al., 2020; Commins, 2020)

1. **Delayed reactions confuse the timeline.** When symptoms appear 3-8 hours after eating, patients rarely connect them to dinner. They blame midnight snacks, stress, or seemingly random triggers.
2. **Inconsistent symptoms muddy the waters.** One person gets hives; another has gastrointestinal distress; a third experiences anaphylaxis. The same person might have different reactions each time. (Croglio et al., 2021; Richards et al., 2022)

3. **Standard allergy tests miss it.** Traditional skin prick tests using commercial meat extracts often show false negatives. Only specific IgE blood tests for alpha-gal antibodies provide reliable results.
4. **Medical education hasn't caught up.** Most medical schools barely mention AGS. Continuing education focuses on common conditions, not emerging syndromes affecting less than 1% of the population.
5. **Geographic bias affects recognition.** Doctors in low-tick areas rarely consider AGS, while physicians in endemic regions might test for it routinely. (Kim et al., 2020; Wilson et al., 2024)

Who Gets AGS? Surprising Risk Patterns

The demographics of AGS shatter stereotypes about who develops allergies. While children commonly develop food allergies, AGS primarily affects adults aged 40-69, with cases reported from age 5 to over 90 (Pattanaik et al., 2018). Men slightly outnumber women, possibly due to greater outdoor exposure, though rates are equalizing as outdoor recreation patterns change. (Thompson et al., 2023; Ailsworth et al., 2024)

Certain blood types appear more susceptible. People with blood types B and AB show lower rates of AGS, possibly because they naturally produce a sugar similar to alpha-gal. Type O and A individuals face higher risk, though scientists still debate the exact mechanisms (Rispens et al., 2022).

Occupational exposure creates clear risk patterns:

- Forestry workers show AGS rates 10 times higher than office workers
- Hunters and outdoor enthusiasts face elevated risk
- Military personnel training in wooded areas report increasing cases (Thompson et al., 2023; Ailsworth et al., 2024)

- Landscapers and golf course workers encounter daily tick exposure (Kim et al., 2020; Wilson et al., 2024)

Yet AGS doesn't discriminate by occupation alone. Weekend gardeners, suburban dog walkers, and children playing in backyards all face potential exposure. The ticks don't care about your job title - they care about finding a blood meal. (Wilson et al., 2019)

The Genetic Wild Card

Emerging research suggests genetic factors influence AGS development. Not everyone bitten by ticks develops the syndrome, even with multiple bites. Studies of families show clustering patterns beyond shared environmental exposure, hinting at hereditary susceptibility (McGinley et al., 2024).

Some people produce more robust IgE responses to alpha-gal, while others mount minimal reactions. Variations in genes controlling antibody production, mast cell sensitivity, and immune regulation all potentially influence who develops AGS after tick exposure. This genetic lottery explains why two hunters in the same deer stand might have vastly different outcomes after identical tick encounters. (Kim et al., 2020; Wilson et al., 2024)

Climate Change and the Expanding Threat

The Lone Star tick's range expansion tells a climate story. These ticks thrive in warm, humid conditions - exactly what climate change delivers to previously cooler regions. Counties reporting established Lone Star tick populations increased by 30% between 2010 and 2022 (Springer et al., 2024). (Kim et al., 2020; Wilson et al., 2024)

Computer models predict continued northward expansion, potentially exposing millions more Americans to AGS risk. By

2050, suitable tick habitat could extend into southern Canada, while current tick-free refuges in the Mountain West might see new invasions. Public health officials in Minnesota, Wisconsin, and Michigan already report increasing AGS cases as tick populations establish themselves. (Thompson et al., 2023; Ailsworth et al., 2024)

But it's not just about geography. Warmer winters mean ticks remain active longer. What used to be a summer risk now extends from March through November in many regions. Mild temperatures accelerate tick life cycles, increasing population density. More ticks plus longer seasons equals exponentially higher exposure risk. (Kim et al., 2020; Wilson et al., 2024)

The Medical Community's Knowledge Crisis

That 42% figure - doctors who've never heard of AGS - represents more than a statistics problem. It's a human tragedy multiplied thousands of times. Every unaware physician potentially sends AGS patients down months or years of diagnostic dead ends. The knowledge gap concentrates in specialties you'd expect to know better: 35% of allergists, 45% of emergency physicians, and 48% of primary care providers report zero familiarity with AGS (Carpenter et al., 2023).

Medical schools compound the problem. A survey of 50 medical school curricula found that only 12% included any mention of AGS, usually buried in broader discussions of tick-borne diseases. Residency programs fare no better - even allergy and immunology fellowships average less than one hour of AGS education across three years of training (Kumar et al., 2024). (Kim et al., 2020; Wilson et al., 2024)

The consequences ripple outward. Undiagnosed patients crowd emergency rooms with preventable reactions. Insurance companies pay for extensive testing that misses the obvious. Patients lose faith in medical systems that can't explain their suffering. Some turn to questionable alternative treatments or simply give up seeking help.

Accelerating Your Own Diagnosis

Knowledge becomes power when navigating medical uncertainty. If you suspect AGS, these strategies can shorten your diagnostic journey:

Document everything meticulously. Create a symptom diary noting:

- Exact times you ate mammalian products
- When symptoms started and peaked
- Specific symptoms and their severity
- What helped (antihistamines, epinephrine, time)
- Activities between eating and symptoms

Use precise medical language. Instead of "I had a reaction," say "I experienced urticaria and angioedema approximately 4 hours after consuming beef." Specific terminology gets attention and suggests you've done homework. (Commins et al., 2009; Commins et al., 2014)

Request specific testing. Ask for "alpha-gal specific IgE blood testing" rather than general allergy panels. Include component testing for beef, pork, lamb, and milk if available. Some labs offer more comprehensive panels than others. (Commins et al., 2009; Commins et al., 2014)

Bring evidence. Print relevant medical journal articles. The CDC's AGS webpage carries weight. Photos of reactions help doubting doctors see what you experience. (CDC, 2025; CDC, 2025)

Consider geographic expertise. If local doctors seem clueless, consider telemedicine consultations with physicians in AGS-endemic areas. Many university medical centers in Virginia, North Carolina, and Tennessee offer remote appointments.

The Hidden Epidemic Revealed

AGS represents more than a medical curiosity - it's a preview of emerging health challenges in our changing world. As environments shift and vectors expand, new diseases emerge at accelerating rates. AGS teaches us that modern medicine must stay nimble, that patient advocacy matters, and that sometimes the most unlikely explanations prove correct.

The syndrome also exposes healthcare disparities. Rural communities with high tick exposure often lack specialty medical care. Lower-income patients can't afford multiple specialist visits chasing diagnosis. Those without internet access miss online AGS communities that could guide them to answers. Geographic knowledge clusters mean identical symptoms receive different responses based on where you seek care. (Platts-Mills et al., 2020; Commins, 2020)

Yet hope emerges from growing awareness. Medical conferences now feature AGS sessions. Journals publish increasing research. Patient advocacy groups spread information faster than traditional medical education. Each diagnosed patient becomes an educator, sharing knowledge with family, friends, and sometimes skeptical doctors.

Key Takeaways from The Hidden Epidemic

The AGS epidemic hides in plain sight, affecting hundreds of thousands while remaining invisible to much of medicine. Understanding these realities empowers your journey:

- AGS affects up to 450,000 Americans, yet 42% of healthcare providers haven't heard of it

- Average diagnosis takes seven years due to delayed reactions, inconsistent symptoms, and medical knowledge gaps (Platts-Mills et al., 2020; Commins, 2020)
- Geographic location strongly influences diagnosis speed - endemic areas recognize AGS faster (Platts-Mills et al., 2020; Commins, 2020)
- Adults 40-69 face highest risk, with outdoor workers and recreationalists especially vulnerable
- Blood type, genetics, and tick exposure patterns all influence AGS development (Kim et al., 2020; Wilson et al., 2024)
- Climate change expands tick ranges, exposing new populations to risk (Kim et al., 2020; Wilson et al., 2024)
- Patient self-advocacy and specific test requests can dramatically shorten diagnosis time (Platts-Mills et al., 2020; Commins, 2020)
- Medical education slowly adapts, but patient communities lead awareness efforts

The hidden epidemic emerges from shadows as more patients find answers, more doctors gain knowledge, and more communities recognize the threat in their backyards. Your awareness might save years of suffering - for yourself or someone you love.

Chapter 2: The Science Made Simple

Your immune system just got hacked by a tick. Not infected, not diseased - hacked, like a computer programmed to attack something that was always safe before. This biological hack turns your body against a sugar molecule that exists in nearly every mammal except you. Understanding how this happens means grasping some science, but don't worry - we'll walk through it together, no PhD required. (Kim et al., 2020; Wilson et al., 2024)

The story starts with evolution. About 20-30 million years ago, our ancestors lost the ability to make a particular sugar called galactose-alpha-1,3-galactose (alpha-gal for short). This genetic change separated us from other mammals - humans, apes, and Old World monkeys stand alone in lacking this sugar (Macher & Galili, 2008). For millions of years, this quirk meant nothing. Our bodies encountered alpha-gal in food and ignored it, just another foreign molecule among thousands we consume daily.

Then certain ticks entered the picture, carrying alpha-gal in their saliva. When these ticks bite, they inject this sugar directly into our bloodstream along with other tick proteins that alert our immune system to danger. Your body, programmed to attack foreign invaders accompanied by danger signals, creates antibodies against alpha-gal. Now you're sensitized - your immune system treats this sugar as a threat wherever it appears, including in the burger you eat next week (Commins & Platts-Mills, 2013). (Kim et al., 2020; Wilson et al., 2024)

The Tick That Changes Everything

Not all ticks trigger AGS. In the United States, the Lone Star tick (*Amblyomma americanum*) bears primary responsibility, though blacklegged ticks and others occasionally contribute. These ticks pick up alpha-gal from feeding on mammals - deer, dogs, cattle, mice. The sugar concentrates in their saliva, ready for injection into the next host (Crispell et al., 2019).

Female Lone Star ticks, identified by the white spot on their backs, feed for 7-10 days, plenty of time to trigger immune sensitization. But here's what's strange - not every Lone Star tick bite causes AGS. Factors like the tick's previous blood meals, how long it feeds, and your individual immune response all matter. Some people endure dozens of bites without developing AGS; others need just one perfectly wrong bite.

The tick's saliva contains more than alpha-gal. Proteins, lipids, and other molecules create an immunological cocktail that essentially tells your body, "Pay attention! Dangerous stuff incoming!" This danger signal, combined with alpha-gal's foreign nature, triggers what immunologists call a perfect storm of sensitization (Cabezas-Cruz et al., 2023).

Your Immune System's Case of Mistaken Identity

To understand AGS, you need to know how allergies work. Your immune system constantly surveys everything entering your body, deciding friend or foe. Usually, it correctly identifies food as harmless. But sometimes wires get crossed, and harmless substances get labeled dangerous.

In typical food allergies, IgE antibodies - think of them as molecular wanted posters - attach to mast cells throughout your body. When the "wanted" food appears, antibodies signal mast cells to release histamine and other chemicals, causing allergic symptoms. This usually happens within minutes because the allergen (like peanut protein) absorbs quickly from your digestive tract (Iweala & Burks, 2016).

AGS breaks these rules. First, alpha-gal is a sugar, not a protein like most food allergens. Second, it's attached to proteins and fats in mammalian meat, which digest slowly. Third, alpha-gal absorbs primarily through your intestines rather than your mouth or stomach. This unique absorption pattern explains the signature delayed reaction of AGS. (Commins et al., 2009; Commins et al., 2014)

The 3-8 Hour Mystery Explained

Picture eating a steak at 6 PM. The meat enters your stomach, where acid and enzymes begin breaking down proteins. But alpha-gal, attached to fats and proteins, resists quick digestion. Your meal moves to the small intestine around 8-9 PM, where bile salts finally start liberating alpha-gal from its attachments (Wilson et al., 2021).

Now free, alpha-gal crosses the intestinal wall into your bloodstream, packaged in particles called chylomicrons - essentially fat droplets that transport dietary lipids. This process peaks 3-5 hours after eating. Your IgE antibodies finally meet their target around 10 PM to midnight, triggering mast cells to release their chemical arsenal. You wake at 1 AM with hives, wondering what hit you.

The delay varies based on several factors:

- **Fat content**: Fattier meats delay absorption further
- **Processing**: Organ meats often trigger faster reactions
- **Individual digestion**: Your personal gut transit time matters
- **Meal composition**: Other foods can speed or slow absorption

This timing makes AGS particularly dangerous. Traditional food allergies strike quickly - you know immediately something's wrong. With AGS, you might be asleep when reactions peak, far from help and confused about the cause. Many patients report waking to find themselves covered in hives or struggling to breathe, with no obvious connection to dinner hours earlier.

Understanding Your Alpha-Gal Numbers

The blood test for AGS measures IgE antibodies specific to alpha-gal, reported in kU/L (kilounits per liter). But interpreting these numbers requires nuance - they're not like pregnancy tests with simple yes/no answers (Commins et al., 2016).

Typical ranges:

- < 0.10 kU/L: Negative
- 0.10 - 0.34 kU/L: Borderline
- 0.35 - 0.70 kU/L: Low positive
- 0.71 - 3.50 kU/L: Moderate positive
- 3.51 - 17.50 kU/L: High positive
- 17.50 kU/L: Very high positive

But here's where it gets complicated - numbers don't perfectly predict reactions. Some people with levels of 0.5 have severe anaphylaxis, while others with levels over 10 eat bacon daily without issues. Your personal threshold depends on multiple factors beyond antibody levels.

Component testing adds clarity by measuring IgE to specific meats: (Macdougall et al., 2022; Apostolovic et al., 2023)

- Beef (Bos d 6)
- Pork (Sus s 1)
- Lamb (Ovis a 1)
- Milk proteins containing alpha-gal

Patterns matter. Someone with high beef IgE but low pork might tolerate bacon but react to steak. Milk numbers help predict dairy tolerance. Trends over time indicate whether sensitivity is increasing or decreasing. (Commins et al., 2009; Commins et al., 2014)

When Perfect Storms Create Severe Reactions

AGS reactions vary wildly, even in the same person. Tuesday's burger causes mild itching; Saturday's leads to emergency treatment. These co-factors can transform minor reactions into major crises:

Exercise tops the danger list. Physical activity increases gut permeability, allowing more alpha-gal absorption. Blood flow changes during exercise also spread allergens faster. Many patients report their worst reactions followed eating plus exercise - the Saturday afternoon golf game after a burger lunch becomes a medical emergency (Brestoff et al., 2017).

Alcohol acts similarly, increasing intestinal permeability and speeding absorption. Beer with barbecue creates double trouble. Wine appears less problematic, though any alcohol potentially worsens reactions. Some patients tolerate meat only with complete alcohol abstinence.

NSAIDs (aspirin, ibuprofen, naproxen) increase gut permeability and amplify immune responses. Taking ibuprofen for post-workout soreness after eating meat creates a triple threat - exercise, NSAIDs, and alpha-gal exposure combined. Many AGS patients must switch to acetaminophen (Fischer et al., 2017).

Tick bites themselves temporarily worsen reactions. Fresh bites boost IgE production and prime mast cells for reactivity. Patients often report increased sensitivity for weeks after new bites, requiring extra dietary caution during tick season.

Stress and illness compromise gut barriers and immune regulation. Major life stress, infections, or chronic conditions can suddenly worsen previously stable AGS. The same meal tolerated during calm periods might trigger reactions during stressful times.

Sleep deprivation affects immune function and gut health. Night shift workers and chronic insomniacs often report increased AGS sensitivity. Regular sleep patterns help maintain consistent reaction thresholds.

The Molecular Mechanics of Misery

Let's go deeper into what happens during an AGS reaction. When alpha-gal-bearing particles enter your bloodstream, they encounter IgE antibodies coating mast cells. These antibodies work like locks waiting for the right key. Alpha-gal provides that key, causing antibodies to cross-link - imagine molecular hands clasping together (Stone et al., 2019).

This cross-linking triggers mast cells to degranulate - basically, explode their contents into surrounding tissue. Within seconds, these cells release:

- **Histamine**: Causes itching, flushing, and blood vessel dilation
- **Tryptase**: Contributes to low blood pressure and shock
- **Leukotrienes**: Trigger airway constriction and mucus production
- **Prostaglandins**: Create pain, fever, and inflammation
- **Cytokines**: Call other immune cells to join the party

The cascade amplifies quickly. One activated mast cell triggers neighbors, creating waves of reaction throughout your body. Blood vessels dilate and leak, causing hives and swelling. Airways constrict. Blood pressure drops. Your body essentially launches nuclear war against a sugar molecule.

Why Some React and Others Don't

The mystery of variable reactions puzzles researchers and frustrates patients. Two people with identical IgE levels eat the same meal - one needs epinephrine, the other feels fine. Several theories explain this variability:

Mast cell burden varies between individuals. Some people naturally have more mast cells or more reactive ones. Conditions like mast cell activation syndrome amplify AGS reactions. Genetics influence mast cell numbers and sensitivity (Carter et al., 2022).

Gut microbiome differences affect alpha-gal processing. Certain bacteria might break down alpha-gal before absorption. Others could enhance absorption or create metabolites that worsen reactions. Antibiotic use, diet changes, and probiotics all potentially impact AGS through microbiome effects.

Hormonal fluctuations influence immune responses. Many women report worse reactions during menstruation or menopause. Thyroid disorders, common in middle age, affect reaction severity. Cortisol patterns - your natural stress hormone - modulate allergic responses throughout the day.

Tissue-specific IgE might explain organ-specific reactions. Some patients only get gut symptoms; others only skin reactions. The distribution and density of armed mast cells in different organs could create these patterns. Your personal mast cell map determines where reactions hit hardest. (Thompson et al., 2023; Ailsworth et al., 2024)

Individual absorption patterns vary based on gut anatomy, transit time, and digestive enzymes. People with faster digestion might absorb alpha-gal differently than slow digesters. Previous gut surgery, inflammatory bowel disease, or even normal aging changes absorption dynamics.

The Glycan Code Your Body Can't Crack

Alpha-gal belongs to a family of molecules called glycans - sugar chains that decorate proteins and fats throughout nature. Your body reads these glycan codes constantly, using them to identify self versus non-self, healthy cells versus damaged ones. Cancer cells change their glycan signatures. Bacteria wear distinctive glycan uniforms. Your immune system evolved as a sophisticated glycan reader (Cummings & Pierce, 2021). (Macdougall et al., 2022; Apostolovic et al., 2023)

But evolution played a trick. When our ancestors lost alpha-gal production, they gained the ability to make antibodies against it. This probably helped fight infections - many pathogens wear alpha-gal. For millions of years, this worked great. Eat a mammoth, digest it completely, no problems. The cooking and digestion destroyed most immunogenic alpha-gal structures.

Modern food processing changed the game. We eat fresher meat, less thoroughly cooked, with alpha-gal structures more intact. Refrigeration, restaurant preparation, and preferences for rare meat all potentially increase alpha-gal exposure compared to our ancestors' thoroughly cooked, often partially spoiled meat consumption.

Cross-Reactions and Unexpected Triggers

AGS antibodies don't just recognize meat. The alpha-gal structure appears in unexpected places, creating surprising reaction triggers:

Mammalian organs concentrate alpha-gal. Kidney, liver, and sweetbreads cause severe reactions even in people who tolerate muscle meat. The organs' rich blood supply and cellular structure pack more alpha-gal per bite. Some patients must avoid organ meat completely while enjoying regular steaks (Mabelane et al., 2018).

Dairy contains alpha-gal attached to proteins and fats. Most AGS patients tolerate dairy initially, but sensitivity often expands over time. The progression typically follows: cream → milk → cheese → butter. Some lucky folks keep dairy tolerance throughout; others lose it all.

Gelatin triggers reactions in sensitive individuals. This means marshmallows, gummy candies, gel-cap medications, and certain vaccines become problems. The rendering process that creates gelatin concentrates alpha-gal from animal bones and skin. (Stone et al., 2017; Zafar et al., 2022)

Mammalian-derived medical products pose serious risks:

- Heparin (blood thinner from pigs)
- Bovine or porcine heart valves
- Surgical mesh from animal collagen
- Certain sutures
- Some vaccines grown in mammalian cells

The Evolution of Individual Reactions

Your AGS doesn't stay static. Like a living thing, it evolves based on exposures, time, and management. Understanding these patterns helps predict your future course: (Platts-Mills et al., 2020; Commins, 2020)

Initial sensitization often starts mild. First reactions might seem like food poisoning or random hives. Each exposure potentially increases sensitivity as your body produces more IgE antibodies. The crescendo builds over months or years until reactions become unmistakable.

Peak sensitivity typically occurs 1-3 years after onset. Your body maximizes antibody production, mast cells stand fully armed, and reactions hit hardest. This period requires strictest avoidance and greatest caution. Many patients need epinephrine prescriptions during peak years (Pattanaik et al., 2020).

Plateau phase follows as reactions stabilize. You learn your triggers, avoid co-factors, and reactions become predictable. Some patients maintain this steady state indefinitely with careful management.

Potential decline offers hope. Without re-exposure to tick bites, many patients see IgE levels fall over 3-5 years. Reactions mild, dietary restrictions loosen, and some achieve complete remission. But this requires absolute tick avoidance - one new bite can restart the entire cycle.

Key Takeaways from The Science Made Simple

Understanding AGS mechanisms empowers better management. These scientific insights translate to practical strategies:

- Alpha-gal is a sugar you can't produce but exists in all mammals you might eat
- Tick saliva programs your immune system to attack this previously harmless molecule
- Reactions delay 3-8 hours because alpha-gal must be digested and absorbed with fats
- IgE blood levels help but don't perfectly predict reaction severity
- Co-factors like exercise, alcohol, and NSAIDs transform mild reactions into emergencies
- Individual variation depends on mast cells, microbiome, hormones, and absorption patterns
- AGS evolves over time - usually worsening initially, potentially improving with tick avoidance
- Cross-reactions extend beyond meat to dairy, gelatin, and medical products (Stone et al., 2017; Zafar et al., 2022)

The science seems complex because it is. AGS breaks traditional allergy rules, creating a new paradigm requiring new understanding. But knowledge brings power - understanding why reactions happen helps predict and prevent them. Your biological hack has patterns, and recognizing those patterns puts you back in control.

Chapter 3: Getting Properly Diagnosed

The medical system failed Jennifer Chen for three years. This software engineer from Austin documented everything meticulously - spreadsheets tracking meals, symptoms, timing, severity. She'd seen two primary care doctors, a gastroenterologist, an allergist, and made four emergency room visits. Total cost: $12,000 and counting. The diagnosis they missed? Alpha-gal syndrome, finally caught by a physician assistant who'd attended a recent conference on tick-borne conditions.

Jennifer's story repeats thousands of times across America. Smart, engaged patients with clear symptoms get shuffled through expensive medical mazes while the obvious answer hides in plain sight. But you don't have to follow this path. Getting properly diagnosed with AGS requires strategy, persistence, and knowing exactly what to ask for (Pattanaik et al., 2018).

Finding Doctors Who Actually Know AGS

Start with geographic advantage. Physicians in tick-endemic areas see more AGS, building real-world expertise beyond textbook knowledge. The University of North Carolina, University of Virginia, Vanderbilt, and Washington University in St. Louis lead AGS research and treatment. Their allergy departments train fellows who spread knowledge nationwide.

But you probably can't travel to these centers. So how do you find local expertise? Start with these strategies:

Search academic medical centers within 200 miles. Teaching hospitals stay more current with emerging conditions. Their physicians attend conferences, read journals, and teach residents about new developments. Call their allergy departments directly - ask if any physicians have AGS experience.

Check AGS support groups for physician recommendations. The Alpha-Gal Support Facebook group (30,000+ members) maintains informal lists of AGS-aware doctors by state. Patients share experiences, warning about dismissive physicians and praising those who listen. Real-world experience beats credentials.

Contact local Lyme disease specialists. Doctors treating tick-borne illnesses often know AGS, even if it's not their primary focus. They understand tick exposure risks and stay current on tick-related conditions. Many diagnosed their first AGS cases by accident while evaluating Lyme patients. (Thompson et al., 2023; Ailsworth et al., 2024)

Use telemedicine strategically. Many AGS experts offer video consultations. While they can't order tests directly in other states, they provide guidance your local doctor can follow. A one-time consultation with an expert often provides the roadmap for local management.

Interview potential doctors before committing. Call and ask: "How many AGS patients do you treat? What's your diagnostic approach? Do you test for component allergens or just total alpha-gal IgE?" Blank silence or defensiveness suggests moving on. Enthusiasm and specific answers indicate potential partnership.

Red flags to avoid:

- "I've never heard of that"
- "Food allergies don't work that way"
- "Maybe it's psychological"
- "Let's try eliminating gluten first"

- "Your tests are negative, so it can't be that"

The Testing Cascade That Actually Works

Proper AGS diagnosis requires specific tests in the right order. Many doctors order wrong tests or interpret results incorrectly. Here's the optimal cascade (Wilson et al., 2019):

Step 1: Alpha-gal specific IgE (the essential test)

- Test name: Galactose-alpha-1,3-galactose (alpha-gal) IgE
- Lab codes: Quest 95241, LabCorp 602665
- Measures: Total antibodies against alpha-gal
- Cost: $100-200 without insurance
- Results time: 3-5 days

This single test diagnoses most AGS cases. Levels above 0.35 kU/L are considered positive, though some laboratories use 0.10 as the cutoff. Request actual numbers, not just positive/negative results. The specific level helps predict severity and guide management.

Step 2: Component testing (for detailed understanding)

- Beef (Bos d 6) IgE
- Pork (Sus s 1) IgE
- Lamb (Ovis a 1) IgE
- Cow's milk IgE
- Cat epithelium IgE (contains alpha-gal)
- Dog dander IgE (cross-reactivity marker)

Component testing reveals individual sensitivities. Someone might react strongly to pork but tolerate beef, or vice versa. This granular data guides dietary choices beyond simple meat avoidance. (Commins et al., 2009; Commins et al., 2014)

Step 3: Baseline tryptase (for reaction severity assessment)

- Measures: Mast cell stability
- Normal range: 2-10 ng/mL
- Elevated baseline suggests higher reaction risk
- Important for emergency planning

Step 4: Complete blood count with eosinophils

- Rules out eosinophilic disorders
- Establishes baseline for monitoring
- May show mild eosinophilia in AGS

Step 5: Comprehensive metabolic panel

- Ensures no organ damage from reactions
- Baseline for medication safety
- Screens for comorbidities

Avoid these common testing mistakes:

- Skin prick tests with commercial meat extracts (often false negative)
- Total IgE only (misses specific alpha-gal antibodies)
- Standard food allergy panels (rarely include alpha-gal)
- ImmunoCAP without specific alpha-gal request
- Testing during antihistamine use (may suppress results)

Documenting Your Case Like a Detective

Doctors respond to data. Vague complaints get vague responses. Build an irrefutable case with systematic documentation:

The AGS Symptom Diary should track:

- **Exact foods eaten** with times, portions, and preparation methods

- **Symptom onset** to the minute when possible
- **Symptom progression** - what appeared first, how it evolved
- **Severity scoring** on a 1-10 scale for each symptom
- **Interventions** - what you took, when, and results
- **Recovery time** - when you felt normal again
- **Co-factors** - exercise, alcohol, medications, stress level
- **Recent tick exposure** - new bites within past month

Create a one-page summary showing:

- Frequency of reactions (X times per month)
- Common triggers with reaction rates
- Average onset time after eating
- Typical symptom progression
- Emergency room visits or medical interventions

Photography proves your point. Pictures of hives, swelling, or rashes provide undeniable evidence. Time-stamp photos showing progression. Include a ruler or coin for scale. Create a photo timeline of a typical reaction.

Bring supporting materials:

- Printouts of major AGS studies
- CDC's AGS information page
- Your detailed symptom diary
- Photo documentation
- List of failed treatments tried
- Questions prepared in advance

Speaking the Medical Language

How you describe symptoms affects how seriously doctors take you. Replace vague terms with medical precision:

Instead of: "I get sick after eating meat" Say: "I experience delayed IgE-mediated reactions 3-6 hours after consuming mammalian products" (Commins et al., 2009; Commins et al., 2014)

Instead of: "I break out in bumps" Say: "I develop generalized urticaria progressing to angioedema"

Instead of: "My stomach hurts" Say: "I have severe cramping abdominal pain with nausea and diarrhea" (Croglio et al., 2021; Richards et al., 2022)

Instead of: "I can't breathe well" Say: "I experience respiratory distress with sensation of throat constriction"

This isn't about impressing anyone - it's about accurate communication that triggers appropriate medical response. Doctors document what you say. Precise language generates precise records, supporting insurance coverage and appropriate treatment.

Navigating Insurance Obstacles

Insurance companies haven't caught up with AGS reality. Many still consider alpha-gal testing "experimental" or "not medically necessary." Fight these denials with strategy (Herman et al., 2023):

Pre-authorization wins battles. Before testing, have your doctor submit:

- Letter of medical necessity
- Documentation of reactions
- Failed alternative diagnoses
- Relevant medical literature
- CPT codes with justification

Proper coding matters:

- ICD-10: Z91.018 (Allergy to other foods)
- Add: W57.XXXA (Bitten by other nonvenomous arthropods)
- Include: T78.00XA (Anaphylactic reaction due to unspecified food)

Appeal denials immediately. Insurance companies count on patient exhaustion. First-level appeals succeed 40% of the time. Include:

- Your symptom documentation
- Photos of reactions
- Doctor's detailed letter
- Published AGS studies
- Cost comparison (testing vs. repeated ER visits)

Track every expense. FSA and HSA funds cover AGS testing and treatment. Maintain records for tax deductions if medical expenses exceed 7.5% of income. Some patients successfully argue for coverage of specialty foods as medical expenses.

Self-pay strategies when insurance fails:

- Direct laboratory ordering (often 50-70% cheaper)
- Cash discounts at hospitals
- Payment plans for larger bills
- Laboratory financial assistance programs
- Clinical trial participation for free testing

When Standard Doctors Strike Out

Sometimes you must bypass traditional channels. These alternatives provide diagnosis when conventional medicine fails:

Functional medicine practitioners often recognize AGS faster. They're trained to investigate root causes of mysterious symptoms. While insurance rarely covers functional medicine, the investment often yields faster diagnosis than years of specialist referrals.

Naturopathic doctors in licensed states can order laboratory tests. Many stay current on environmental illness trends. They spend more time with patients, increasing chances of connecting dietary dots.

Direct laboratory testing in available states lets you order tests yourself. Companies like Walk-In Lab, Ulta Lab Tests, and others offer alpha-gal panels. Results go directly to you for interpretation or sharing with doctors.

Clinical trials sometimes offer free testing. Search ClinicalTrials.gov for AGS studies. Participants receive expert evaluation and contribute to research. Major centers regularly recruit for various AGS investigations.

Building Your Medical Team

AGS management requires more than one doctor. Build a comprehensive team:

Primary care physician coordinates overall care, manages prescriptions, and provides referrals. Find one willing to learn about AGS even if initially unfamiliar. Teachable beats know-it-all.

Allergist/immunologist manages testing, monitors IgE trends, and prescribes emergency medications. Ideally, find one with AGS experience, but any good allergist can learn current protocols.

Registered dietitian helps navigate nutritional challenges. Look for experience with elimination diets and food allergies. Many offer telehealth consultations specifically for AGS patients.

Mental health support addresses anxiety and lifestyle adjustments. Chronic illness takes psychological tolls. Therapists experienced with medical trauma and dietary restrictions provide valuable support.

Emergency medicine awareness saves lives. Provide your local ER with AGS information. Meet with the medical director if possible. Ensure they stock appropriate medications and understand delayed reaction patterns.

The Diagnosis Day Game Plan

When you finally see an AGS-aware doctor, maximize the appointment:

Arrive prepared with organized documentation, questions listed by priority, and realistic expectations. Bring support person to take notes and advocate if needed.

Start with impact: "I've had 15 delayed reactions to meat over six months, documented here, and I need alpha-gal testing to confirm suspected AGS."

Present evidence efficiently. Hand over your one-page summary. Offer detailed documentation if requested. Show photos on your phone rather than printing everything.

Ask specific questions:

- What's your AGS testing protocol?
- How do you interpret borderline results?
- Will you prescribe epinephrine today?
- Can we schedule follow-up testing in 6 months?

- Do you have AGS dietary resources?

Request immediate needs:

- Alpha-gal IgE testing order
- Epinephrine prescription (don't leave without it)
- Medical alert bracelet prescription (insurance coverage)
- Work/school accommodation letter if needed
- Referrals to other team members

Confirm next steps before leaving. When will results arrive? How will they be communicated? What constitutes an emergency? When should you follow up?

Key Takeaways from Getting Properly Diagnosed

Navigating AGS diagnosis requires persistence and strategy. These approaches accelerate your journey:

- Geographic location affects physician awareness - seek doctors in tick-endemic areas or via telemedicine
- Specific testing cascade starts with alpha-gal IgE, then components, baseline tryptase
- Detailed documentation with photos and precise medical language strengthens your case
- Insurance obstacles require pre-authorization, proper coding, and determined appeals
- Alternative routes include functional medicine, direct testing, and clinical trials when traditional medicine fails
- Building a complete medical team ensures comprehensive care beyond diagnosis
- Prepared patients presenting organized evidence receive faster, more accurate diagnosis
- Emergency medications like epinephrine should be prescribed immediately upon AGS confirmation

The path to proper AGS diagnosis shouldn't take seven years. Armed with knowledge, documentation, and determination, you can compress that timeline to weeks or months. The key lies in becoming your own advocate, speaking medicine's language, and refusing to accept "we don't know" as a final answer. Your symptoms are real, your condition has a name, and proper diagnosis opens the door to reclaiming your life.

Chapter 4: The First 30 Days

The diagnosis hit Marcus Rodriguez like a freight train on Tuesday. By Wednesday morning, he stood in his kitchen at 6 AM, staring at his refrigerator like it had betrayed him. Twenty years of morning routines - bacon and eggs, leftover pizza, ham sandwiches for lunch - suddenly felt like navigating a minefield. His wife found him there an hour later, still holding the door open, paralyzed by the simple question of what to eat for breakfast.

"I kept thinking someone would hand me a manual," Marcus told me later. "You know, 'Congratulations, you have AGS, here's exactly what to do.' Instead, I got a two-minute explanation, an EpiPen prescription, and a cheerful 'avoid mammalian meat!' Like that means anything when you're standing in your kitchen wondering if butter will kill you." (Commins et al., 2009; Commins et al., 2014)

Those first 30 days after AGS diagnosis often determine your entire trajectory. Handle them well, and you build a foundation for manageable life. Fumble through in panic and confusion, and you risk unnecessary reactions, malnutrition, and psychological trauma that takes years to overcome. The difference? Having a clear action plan instead of figuring it out through trial and error - or worse, through emergency room visits.

Your Life Just Changed - Now What?

First, breathe. Seriously. That tightness in your chest right now? Probably anxiety, not an allergic reaction. AGS throws your nervous system into overdrive, making you question every sensation. Is that normal stomach gurgling or the start of a reaction? Was that throat clearing always there, or is your airway closing? This hypervigilance exhausts you, but it's temporary. Your body needs time to recalibrate its alarm system.

33

The most dangerous mistake in these first weeks is overconfidence. "I'll just avoid red meat" sounds simple until you realize alpha-gal hides everywhere. The second most dangerous mistake? Complete paralysis - eating nothing but rice and vegetables because everything else seems risky. Both extremes cause problems. You need a methodical middle path (Commins et al., 2016). (Commins et al., 2009; Commins et al., 2014)

Start with this truth: You're not starting from zero. You've kept yourself alive for decades. You know how to read labels, cook meals, take medications. AGS doesn't erase these skills - it just requires updating them. Think software upgrade, not complete system replacement.

Building Your Emergency Action Plan

Before you eat another meal, before you sort through your pantry, before anything else - create your emergency action plan. This isn't paranoia; it's preparation. The average AGS patient has their worst reaction within the first six months, often because they didn't know what they were dealing with (Wilson et al., 2021).

Your emergency plan needs five components:

1. Recognition criteria - Write down YOUR specific early warning signs. Not textbook symptoms, but your personal pattern. Maybe your ears itch first. Maybe you get suddenly exhausted. Maybe your stomach makes a particular grinding sound. These early warnings give you precious time to intervene.

Maria Chen discovered her tell accidentally: "My tongue feels fizzy, like I licked a battery. Happens about 30 minutes before visible symptoms. That fizzy feeling has saved me from three severe reactions because I could take Benadryl early."

2. Medication protocol - List exactly what to take and when:

- First signs: 50mg diphenhydramine (Benadryl)
- If progressing: Add 20mg cetirizine (Zyrtec)
- Breathing issues or swelling: EpiPen immediately
- After EpiPen: Call 911, second EpiPen ready

Keep this protocol everywhere - wallet, phone, kitchen, car, office. Laminate it. During reactions, your brain fog makes remembering impossible.

3. Emergency contacts in order:

- 911 (seems obvious, but people forget)
- Your spouse/emergency contact
- Your allergist's emergency line
- Local hospital (pre-register if possible)
- Backup person who can drive you

4. Hospital communication card stating: "I have Alpha-Gal Syndrome - severe delayed allergy to mammalian products. Reactions occur 3-8 hours after ingestion. This is IgE-mediated anaphylaxis. Please check all medications for mammalian-derived ingredients including gelatin, glycerin, magnesium stearate, and lactose. Heparin is contraindicated unless no alternatives exist." (Commins et al., 2009; Commins et al., 2014)

5. Recovery tracking - Document what happens AFTER reactions. How long until you feel normal? What helped? What made it worse? This data helps predict and manage future episodes.

The Great Kitchen Purge

Now for the kitchen. This feels overwhelming because it is. You're essentially conducting a forensic investigation of your entire food supply. But here's the thing - you only have to do this once. Well, mostly once. Okay, you'll probably do it three times as you learn more, but the first pass catches the obvious dangers.

Start with a box labeled "DEFINITELY UNSAFE" and another labeled "RESEARCH NEEDED." The third box? "DEFINITELY SAFE." That third box starts empty but fills faster than you'd think.

Obvious removals (straight to unsafe box):

- All beef, pork, lamb, venison, rabbit, goat (Commins et al., 2009; Commins et al., 2014)
- Bacon, ham, pepperoni, salami, hot dogs
- Lard, tallow, beef or pork gelatin
- Soup bases with meat
- Gravies and meat sauces

Requires investigation (research box):

- Seasoning mixes (may contain beef/pork)
- Packaged foods with "natural flavors"
- Vitamins and supplements
- Protein bars and shakes
- Anything with glycerin or gelatin

Check every label for:

- Mammalian meat (obvious)
- Gelatin (unless specified fish or plant-based) (Stone et al., 2017; Zafar et al., 2022)
- Glycerin/Glycerol (unless specified vegetable)
- Lactic acid (usually safe but verify source)
- Lactose (in medications mainly)
- "Natural flavors" (call manufacturer)
- Carrageenan (controversial - some react)
- Rennet (in some cheeses)

Here's where people mess up - they trust front labels. "Vegetable soup" might contain beef broth. "Chicken flavored" rice might use pork enzymes. That healthy smoothie powder? Beef collagen. Read EVERY ingredient, EVERY time. (Commins et al., 2009; Commins et al., 2014)

The Bathroom Medicine Cabinet Audit

That 92% statistic about medication changes? It's real, and it's terrifying. Your bathroom cabinet probably contains multiple alpha-gal sources. This audit saves lives - literally (Muglia et al., 2022).

Immediate medication threats:

- Gel caps (almost always bovine/porcine gelatin) (Hawkins et al., 2020; Nwamara et al., 2022)
- Coated tablets (may contain gelatin)
- Gummy vitamins (mammalian gelatin)
- Some liquid medications (glycerin base)
- Suppositories (often contain gelatin)
- Certain inhalers (lactose carrier)

Check EVERY medication for:

- Active ingredients (rarely problematic)
- Inactive ingredients (the danger zone)
- Coating composition
- Capsule material
- Binding agents

Common problematic inactive ingredients:

- Gelatin (capsules and coatings)
- Magnesium stearate (can be bovine-derived) (Hawkins et al., 2020; Nwamara et al., 2022)
- Lactose (filler in many pills)

- Glycerin (liquid medications)
- Stearic acid (sometimes animal-derived)

Don't stop taking prescribed medications! Instead, contact your pharmacist and doctor immediately. Most medications have safe alternatives. Your pharmacist can research specific manufacturers and find alpha-gal-free versions. This process takes time - start immediately.

Creating Your Safe Food Foundation

Panic makes people eat nothing but salad for weeks. Don't. You need balanced nutrition to heal and maintain energy. Build your safe food foundation methodically:

Proteins you CAN eat:

- Chicken (all forms)
- Turkey (including ground)
- Duck and other poultry
- All fish and seafood
- Eggs (fantastic protein source)
- Plant proteins (beans, lentils, tofu)
- Nuts and seeds
- Protein powders (verify ingredients)

Safe cooking fats:

- Olive oil
- Vegetable oils
- Coconut oil
- Poultry fat (chicken schmaltz)
- Plant-based butter alternatives
- Fish oil

Reliable carbohydrates:

- Rice (all varieties)
- Potatoes (all varieties)
- Pasta (check for egg noodles with milk)
- Bread (verify no milk/butter)
- Oats and cereals (check additives)
- Fruits (all safe)
- Vegetables (all safe)

Initially safe dairy (monitor reactions):

- Hard aged cheeses (lowest alpha-gal)
- Butter (very low alpha-gal)
- Yogurt (moderate levels)
- Milk (higher levels - many react)
- Ice cream (highest levels)

Start a food diary immediately. Not forever - just these first 30 days. Track:

- What you ate (brands matter)
- When you ate it
- Any symptoms (even minor)
- Activities after eating
- Sleep quality
- Energy levels

This diary becomes your personal safety manual. Patterns emerge quickly. Maybe you tolerate cheese but not milk. Maybe exercise after eating triggers reactions. Maybe certain brands work better. Your body teaches you, but only if you're paying attention.

The Psychological Tsunami Nobody Mentions

Here's what the medical literature barely touches - the mental impact of AGS diagnosis. You're grieving. Not just bacon or burgers, but spontaneity, cultural traditions, social ease. That's real loss, and it hits hard.

Common emotional stages in the first 30 days:

Denial - "Maybe it's not that bad. Maybe I'm the exception."
Anger - "This is bulls***! Why me? Stupid ticks!" **Bargaining** - "Maybe just a tiny bit of bacon won't hurt..." **Depression** - "I'll never enjoy food again. Life sucks." **Acceptance** - "Okay, this is my reality. Now what?"

You'll cycle through these repeatedly, sometimes within hours. That's normal. What helps:

- Connect with other AGS patients online
- Allow yourself to feel the feelings
- Focus on what you CAN eat, not restrictions
- Plan one small daily pleasure unrelated to food
- Get professional support if depression persists

Your Daily Routine Reconstruction

Every meal needs rethinking. Start with breakfast - often the hardest meal to reimagine. Common AGS-safe breakfasts:

- Eggs any style with turkey bacon
- Oatmeal with fruits and nuts
- Chicken sausage with potatoes
- Smoothies with plant-based protein
- Avocado toast (check bread)
- Fish (yes, for breakfast - try it)

Lunch strategies:

- Batch cook safe proteins on Sundays
- Keep emergency meals at work
- Research nearby restaurants in advance

- Pack extras - hunger makes you careless
- Have backup snacks always available

Dinner planning:

- Convert favorite recipes using poultry
- Explore international cuisines (many Asian dishes naturally AGS-safe)
- Invest in a good chicken cookbook
- Learn to love seafood if you didn't before
- Make vegetables the star, protein the support

Restaurant Navigation Boot Camp

Eating out feels impossible initially. It's not, but it requires new skills. Your first restaurant meal post-diagnosis should be:

- Somewhere familiar
- During off-peak hours
- With understanding companions
- After calling ahead
- With backup food in your car

Scripts that work: "I have a severe allergy to all mammalian meats including beef, pork, and lamb. I also react to foods cooked on the same surfaces. Can you accommodate this safely?"

If they hesitate even slightly, leave. Seriously. No meal is worth anaphylaxis.

Safe restaurant bets:

- Sushi restaurants (naturally mammal-free)
- Seafood specialists
- Vegetarian/vegan places
- Mediterranean (lots of chicken/fish options)

- Breakfast spots (eggs and poultry)

The Support System Setup

AGS affects everyone around you. Set them up for success:

Immediate family needs:

- Basic AGS education
- Emergency plan familiarity
- List of safe/unsafe foods
- Practice using EpiPen trainer
- Understanding of delayed reactions

Extended family/friends benefit from:

- Simple explanation card
- Your dietary needs for gatherings
- Reassurance you're not being "difficult"
- Specific brands you can eat
- Ways they can help

Workplace modifications:

- Inform HR about your condition
- Update emergency contact information
- Educate close coworkers
- Modify food-related events
- Keep safe snacks in your workspace

Building Your New Normal

By day 30, certain patterns should emerge. You'll know:

- Your safe food staples
- Which restaurants work
- Your early warning signs

- How medications affect you
- Who supports you best

This isn't your final system - it's version 1.0. You'll refine continuously. But having ANY system beats chaos.

Robert Thompson, diagnosed five years ago, told me: "Those first 30 days felt like being dropped in a foreign country where I didn't speak the language and all the food might kill me. But day by day, word by word, meal by meal, I learned. Now it's just life. Different than before, but still good life."

Key Lessons from The First 30 Days

Your AGS journey starts with these crucial first weeks. Master these fundamentals:

- Emergency planning comes first - before eating, before sorting food, before anything
- Kitchen audits require detective-level investigation of every ingredient
- That 92% medication change statistic includes you - audit everything you swallow
- Safe proteins exist abundantly - chicken, turkey, fish, eggs, plants provide complete nutrition
- Emotional chaos is normal - grief, anger, fear all make sense
- Restaurant dining requires new skills but remains entirely possible
- Support systems need education to help effectively
- Version 1.0 of your management system just needs to work, not be perfect

The first 30 days feel impossible because you're building new neural pathways, new habits, new reflexes. Your brain resists this much change. But thousands before you have navigated these waters successfully. Their secret? Taking it one day, one meal, one decision at a time. Tomorrow will be easier than today. Next week easier than this week. In 30 days, you'll look back amazed at how far you've traveled.

Chapter 5: Hidden Dangers Everywhere

Sarah Williams thought she had AGS figured out. Six months post-diagnosis, she'd eliminated all mammalian meat, navigated restaurants successfully, and hadn't had a reaction in weeks. Then came her daughter's birthday party. The cake was safe - she'd checked every ingredient. The ice cream was dairy-free. Even the candy was verified gelatin-free. But three hours later, she found herself in the emergency room, fighting for breath. The culprit? The shiny glaze on the birthday candles contained beef-derived stearic acid.

"I felt so stupid," Sarah told me later. "Who thinks to check birthday candles? But that's the thing with AGS - alpha-gal hides in places you'd never imagine. It's like playing three-dimensional chess when everyone else is playing checkers."

Welcome to the maddening reality of alpha-gal syndrome: the allergen you're avoiding exists in at least 127 documented non-food products, with new sources discovered regularly. From the pills that should heal you to the soap that should clean you, mammalian derivatives infiltrate modern life so thoroughly that complete avoidance becomes nearly impossible. But nearly impossible doesn't mean impossible - it means you need to become a detective (Fischer et al., 2023).

The Pharmaceutical Minefield

Let's start with medications, because this is where hidden alpha-gal can literally threaten your life. You'd think medicines designed to help wouldn't hurt, but the pharmaceutical industry loves mammalian-derived ingredients. They're cheap, effective, and traditionally considered hypoallergenic. Nobody told them about AGS patients.

Gelatin capsules top the danger list. About 90% of capsule medications use either bovine (cow) or porcine (pig) gelatin. That includes: (Hawkins et al., 2020; Nwamara et al., 2022)

- Most antibiotics in capsule form
- Pain medications like Tylenol Arthritis
- Many antidepressants and anxiety medications
- Vitamin D supplements (ironically often prescribed for AGS patients)
- Fish oil supplements (yes, even fish oil often comes in mammalian capsules)
- Probiotics (which you might need due to AGS)

The solution isn't stopping medications - it's finding alternatives. Every capsule medication has either a tablet form, liquid version, or vegetarian capsule option. Your pharmacist can help, but you must specifically request "no mammalian-derived ingredients including gelatin capsules." (Stone et al., 2017; Zafar et al., 2022)

Magnesium stearate, a common tablet lubricant, presents another challenge. While often plant-derived, about 30% comes from beef tallow. Manufacturers rarely specify the source. This ingredient appears in:

- Blood pressure medications
- Cholesterol drugs
- Diabetes medications
- Most vitamins
- Many generic drugs (cheaper to produce with animal-derived stearates)

Lactose as a filler catches many AGS patients off-guard. While lactose itself contains minimal alpha-gal, sensitive individuals react to trace amounts. Common medications with lactose:

- Birth control pills

- Thyroid medications
- Many inhalers
- Some antihistamines
- Various prescription tablets

But wait - there's more hidden pharmaceutical dangers:

Heparin (blood thinner) - derived from pig intestines. Life-threatening for AGS patients. Alternatives exist but must be specifically requested before surgery. (Hawkins et al., 2020; Nwamara et al., 2022)

Pancreatic enzymes - from pigs. People with digestive issues might be prescribed these without knowing the source.

Some vaccines - grown in mammalian cell cultures or containing gelatin stabilizers. Most vaccines have safe alternatives, but you must ask. (Stone et al., 2017; Zafar et al., 2022)

Coated tablets - enteric coatings often contain gelatin. Time-release medications particularly problematic. (Stone et al., 2017; Zafar et al., 2022)

Medical devices also harbor alpha-gal:

- Surgical mesh (often bovine or porcine collagen) (Hawkins et al., 2020; Nwamara et al., 2022)
- Heart valves (pig or cow tissue)
- Surgical sutures (gut sutures from sheep intestines)
- Some wound dressings
- Certain dental implants

Your Personal Care Product Investigation

Now for the bathroom cabinet beyond medications. The personal care industry views animal derivatives as natural, sustainable ingredients. They're everywhere.

Glycerin/Glycerol appears in nearly everything moist:

- Toothpaste (almost all major brands)
- Mouthwash
- Shampoo and conditioner
- Body wash and soap
- Moisturizers and lotions
- Deodorants
- Shaving cream
- Makeup removers

While glycerin CAN be plant-derived, most isn't. Unless the label specifically says "vegetable glycerin," assume animal origin. One AGS patient discovered her severe morning reactions came from toothpaste - she was essentially eating alpha-gal twice daily.

Lanolin (from sheep) triggers reactions in sensitive patients:

- Lip balms and chapsticks
- Nipple creams for nursing
- Heavy moisturizers
- Some sunscreens
- Hair treatments
- Diaper creams

Collagen (usually bovine) shows up in:

- Anti-aging creams
- Hair treatments
- Nail strengtheners
- Some "plumping" lip products
- Sheet masks

- High-end serums

Stearic acid and derivatives hide under multiple names:

- Sodium stearate
- Stearyl alcohol
- Cetearyl alcohol
- Glyceryl stearate
- PEG stearates

These appear in almost every creamy product. Unless certified vegan, assume animal origin.

Other problematic ingredients:

- Tallow (beef fat) in traditional soaps
- Keratin treatments (usually from hooves/horns)
- Elastin (from cow ligaments)
- Carmine/cochineal (red dye from insects - some AGS patients react)
- Emu oil (triggers reactions in many)
- Squalene (can be from sharks)

The Makeup Minefield

Cosmetics present special challenges because they're poorly regulated and incompletely labeled. "Trade secret" protections mean companies don't have to disclose all ingredients.

Common alpha-gal sources in makeup:

- Lipstick (lanolin, carmine, glycerin)
- Foundation (glycerin, stearates)
- Mascara (beeswax, glycerin)
- Eyeshadow (carmine, talc processed with stearates)
- Blush (carmine, lanolin)
- Setting sprays (glycerin)

One patient traced her facial swelling to a high-end foundation containing "marine collagen" - which turned out to be processed with bovine enzymes. Another discovered her lip plumping gloss contained beef collagen. The reactions were mild but constant, creating chronic inflammation she'd attributed to "sensitive skin."

Safe cosmetic strategies:

- Choose explicitly vegan brands
- Research each product before purchasing
- Email companies about specific ingredients
- Patch test everything new
- Keep reaction diary for products
- Build a safe product list slowly

The Cross-Contamination Crisis

Even when you choose safe foods, cross-contamination creates danger. Shared cooking surfaces transfer enough alpha-gal to trigger reactions in sensitive individuals.

Restaurant contamination sources:

- Grills used for both beef and chicken
- Fryers where beef products were cooked
- Cutting boards without proper separation
- Utensils moving between dishes
- Steam tables where juices mingle
- Shared oil for cooking

Michael Johnson learned this painfully: "I ordered grilled chicken at my favorite restaurant. Watched them clean the grill first. Still had a reaction. Turns out, they'd grilled bacon that morning, and the grease had seasoned the grill surface. No amount of scraping removed it completely."

Home kitchen contamination:

- Cast iron pans (absorb and release fats)
- Wooden cutting boards (porous)
- Grills (fat residue in crevices)
- Deep fryers (oil contamination)
- Dishwashers (protein residue)
- Sponges and dish cloths

Solutions for home safety:

- Separate cutting boards (color-coded)
- Dedicated AGS-safe cookware
- Wash contaminated items separately
- Use disposable items when sharing kitchen
- Replace wooden utensils with silicone
- Deep clean everything initially

The Supplement Surprise

Health-conscious AGS patients often turn to supplements, only to discover they're swallowing alpha-gal daily. The supplement industry particularly loves animal-derived ingredients for their bioavailability and low cost.

Problematic supplements:

- Glucosamine (often from shellfish AND beef)
- Chondroitin (from cow cartilage)
- Collagen supplements (obviously)
- Some omega-3s (in gelatin capsules)
- Vitamin D3 (often from lanolin)
- Some probiotics (grown on dairy media)
- Digestive enzymes (from pig pancreas)
- Glandular supplements (organ extracts)

Hidden sources in "vegetarian" supplements:

- Capsules (check for plant-based)
- Flowing agents (magnesium stearate)
- Coatings (may contain gelatin)
- Vitamin D3 (usually animal-derived even in vegan products)

Always verify:

- Capsule material specifically
- All inactive ingredients
- Manufacturing processes
- Shared equipment disclaimers
- Third-party certifications

Pet Products and Household Dangers

Your environment contains surprising alpha-gal sources that create ongoing exposure:

Pet-related exposures:

- Dog food containing beef/pork
- Cat food (almost always mammalian)
- Pet treats and chews
- Rawhide bones
- Pet medications in your home
- Slobber from pets eating meat

Many AGS patients must switch pets to poultry-based foods or accept careful hygiene measures. One patient's mysterious daily hives resolved when she stopped letting her dog lick her face after meals.

Household products with alpha-gal:

- Some laundry detergents (enzymes)
- Fabric softeners (tallow derivatives)

- Bar soaps (sodium tallowate)
- Dishwashing liquids (glycerin)
- All-purpose cleaners (various derivatives)
- Air fresheners (glycerin carriers)
- Dryer sheets (fatty acid derivatives)

Garden and outdoor exposures:

- Fertilizers (bone meal, blood meal)
- Some pesticides (stearate carriers)
- Leather gardening gloves
- Some mulches (processed with animal products)

The Airborne Assault

Yes, you can react to alpha-gal in the air. Cooking fumes carry proteins that trigger sensitive individuals. Problematic scenarios:

Direct cooking exposures:

- Bacon frying (worst offender)
- Grilling meat
- Slow cooker beef stews
- Soup stocks simmering
- Rendering fats
- Barbecue restaurants

Linda Patterson's story: "I walked into my office break room and immediately felt my throat tightening. Someone was microwaving leftover meatloaf. I had to use my inhaler and leave the building. Now I eat lunch in my car."

Indirect airborne exposures:

- Shared ventilation systems
- Clothing carrying cooking odors
- Hair absorbing meat smoke

- Furniture in restaurants
- Car interiors after drive-throughs

Protective strategies:

- Avoid peak restaurant hours
- Request different break room times
- Use personal air purifiers
- Wear masks in high-risk areas
- Shower after exposures
- Change clothing if contaminated

The Social Situation Navigation

Hidden dangers multiply in social settings where you don't control the environment:

Potlucks and parties:

- Serving utensils moving between dishes
- Unknown ingredients in homemade items
- Well-meaning friends who "just used a little bacon"
- Desserts with hidden gelatin
- Drinks with cream liqueurs

Travel exposures:

- Hotel soaps and shampoos
- Restaurant breakfasts (shared griddles)
- Airplane meals (assume contamination)
- Rental car air fresheners
- Laundry services using standard detergents

Workplace hazards:

- Shared microwaves
- Coffee makers with cream residue

- Office celebrations with food
- Business dinners
- Conference meals

Building Your Detection Skills

Becoming an alpha-gal detective requires developing new instincts:

Label reading mastery:

- Read everything, every time
- Learn ingredient synonyms
- Question vague terms
- Verify "natural flavors"
- Check for formula changes
- Save photos of safe products

Key phrases that hide alpha-gal:

- "Natural moisturizing factors"
- "Hydrolyzed proteins"
- "Amino acid complex"
- "Vitamin enriched" (which vitamins?)
- "Time-release coating"
- "Pharmaceutical glaze"

Questions that get answers:

1. "What is the source of your glycerin/gelatin/stearates?" (Stone et al., 2017; Zafar et al., 2022)
2. "Do you use dedicated equipment for vegetarian products?"
3. "Can you provide a complete ingredient list including processing aids?"
4. "Has your formula changed in the last year?"
5. "What carrier do you use for your fragrances?"

Creating Your Safe Zone

Despite these hidden dangers, you can create largely safe environments:

Bathroom sanctuary:

- Curate verified safe products
- Label everything clearly
- Keep backups of favorites
- Store separately from family items
- Document what works

Kitchen confidence:

- Establish contamination-free zones
- Use physical barriers (foil, parchment)
- Implement strict cleaning protocols
- Train family members thoroughly
- Keep emergency supplies visible

Personal protection kit:

- Safe hand soap
- Verified medications
- Emergency snacks
- Barrier supplies (gloves, masks)
- Documentation cards

Key Insights About Hidden Alpha-Gal

The 127 documented sources are just the beginning. New ones emerge constantly as patients react to previously "safe" items. But knowledge empowers protection:

- Pharmaceutical gelatin capsules affect 90% of medications - always request alternatives (Stone et al., 2017; Zafar et al., 2022)
- Personal care glycerin comes from animals unless specifically labeled vegetable-derived
- Cross-contamination on shared surfaces triggers reactions even with "safe" foods
- Airborne proteins from cooking meat can cause respiratory reactions
- Pet products create ongoing home exposure requiring careful management
- Supplements marketed as healthy often contain concentrated animal derivatives
- Social situations multiply hidden exposures through shared utensils and surfaces
- Label reading becomes a survival skill requiring constant vigilance

The hidden dangers feel overwhelming initially. But like learning a new language, pattern recognition develops. You'll start sensing risk, questioning automatically, protecting instinctively. The hypervigilance exhausts you at first but evolves into calm competence. Those 127 sources? They're not hiding anymore - you know where to look.

Chapter 6: Emergency Preparedness

The reaction started at 11:47 PM. David Chen knew because he'd glanced at his phone right before the first wave of nausea hit. By midnight, hives covered his chest. 12:15 AM brought the throat tightness. At 12:22 AM, his wife called 911 while David fumbled with his EpiPen, hands shaking too badly to remove the safety cap. The paramedics arrived at 12:31 AM to find him on the bathroom floor, conscious but struggling, his unused EpiPen still in its case.

"I knew something was wrong," David told me later from his hospital bed. "But my brain kept saying 'wait and see, don't overreact.' By the time I accepted this was anaphylaxis, I could barely think straight. Every second I delayed made the next decision harder."

David's story illustrates emergency preparedness's brutal truth: reactions don't wait for convenient timing or clear thinking. They strike when you're sleeping, driving, alone, or convinced it's just anxiety. The difference between a close call and tragedy often comes down to preparation made when your mind is clear, not decisions made when histamine floods your system (Turner et al., 2022).

Reading Your Body's Secret Messages

Your body whispers before it screams. Learning to hear those whispers can mean the difference between popping a Benadryl at home versus fighting for your life in an ambulance. But here's the challenge - AGS reactions vary wildly between people and even between your own episodes.

Classic AGS warning signs often follow a pattern, though yours might differ:

The 3-4 hour mark (early warnings):

- Sudden fatigue ("I could fall asleep standing up")
- Metallic taste or tingling tongue
- Unexplained anxiety or sense of doom
- Stomach making unusual sounds
- Hot flash or sudden sweating
- Itchy palms or foot soles

The 4-5 hour mark (escalation):

- Visible hives starting (often chest/trunk first)
- Stomach cramping intensifying
- Feeling "not right" or spacey
- Throat clearing repeatedly
- Nose suddenly running
- Heart rate increasing

The 5-6 hour mark (danger zone):

- Hives spreading rapidly
- Swelling of lips, tongue, or face
- Difficulty swallowing
- Wheezing or shortness of breath
- Severe abdominal pain
- Blood pressure dropping (dizziness)

But AGS breaks rules. Sometimes reactions start at 2 hours or wait until 8. Sometimes you skip straight to severe symptoms. Sometimes the usual pattern reverses. This unpredictability means you can't rely on past reactions to predict future ones.

Jennifer Martinez learned this terrifyingly: "My first five reactions were just hives and stomach pain. Annoying but manageable. The sixth time? Full anaphylaxis at hour seven while I was sleeping. If my daughter hadn't heard me wheezing..."

The Medication Hierarchy

When reactions begin, medication timing matters as much as medication choice. Here's your escalation ladder:

First signs - Antihistamine time:

- Diphenhydramine (Benadryl) 50mg - fastest acting
- Cetirizine (Zyrtec) 20mg - longer lasting
- Both together for stubborn symptoms
- Liquid forms work faster than pills
- Chewables beat tablets for speed

Antihistamines work best EARLY. Once massive histamine release occurs, they're like bringing a garden hose to a house fire. Still helpful, but insufficient alone.

Progression despite antihistamines - Support measures:

- Famotidine (Pepcid) 40mg - H2 blocker for gut symptoms
- Albuterol inhaler - if prescribed for breathing
- Prednisone - if prescribed for inflammation
- Zofran - for severe nausea
- Position yourself for potential unconsciousness

The EpiPen decision - Clear criteria:

Use epinephrine immediately for:

- Any breathing difficulty
- Swelling of tongue or throat
- Rapid pulse with dizziness

- Sense of "impending doom"
- Severe symptoms in two or more body systems
- Previous severe reactions with similar start

Don't wait for complete airway closure. Don't debate whether it's "bad enough." Don't worry about wasting it. Delayed epinephrine is the single biggest factor in fatal anaphylaxis outcomes (Kim et al., 2023).

EpiPen technique that works:

1. Remove from case immediately when considering use
2. Blue to the sky, orange to the thigh
3. Swing and push hard through clothing
4. Hold for full 10 seconds (count out loud)
5. Massage injection site for 10 seconds
6. Note the time for paramedics
7. Prepare second pen immediately

After EpiPen - The crucial steps:

- Call 911 immediately (epinephrine can wear off)
- Lie flat with legs elevated (unless vomiting)
- Take photos of symptoms for ER doctors
- List everything eaten in last 8 hours
- Stay warm (shock drops body temperature)
- Keep talking (monitors consciousness)

The ER Reality Check

Emergency rooms save lives but often misunderstand AGS. You might encounter:

- Staff who've never heard of AGS
- Skepticism about delayed reactions
- Pressure to discharge too early
- Medications containing alpha-gal

- Confusion about ongoing symptoms

Prepare for this reality:

Bring documentation:

- Your AGS diagnosis papers
- Allergy action plan from your doctor
- Photos of previous reactions
- List of safe/unsafe medications
- This book's ER information page

Key phrases that get attention: "I have documented IgE-mediated anaphylaxis to galactose-alpha-1,3-galactose. This is a delayed reaction that can biphasic. I need monitoring for at least 4-6 hours after epinephrine."

Demand appropriate treatment:

- IV access maintained
- Continuous monitoring
- H1 and H2 blockers
- Steroid administration
- Verification of all medication ingredients
- Appropriate observation period

Watch for these ER medication dangers:

- Heparin (standard protocol, but dangerous for AGS) (Hawkins et al., 2020; Nwamara et al., 2022)
- Gelatin-containing IV medications
- Lactose-containing pills
- Magnesium stearate in tablets
- Any "standard protocols" without ingredient checks

Susan Thompson's ER experience: "The nurse rolled her eyes when I asked about medication ingredients. Twenty minutes later, I'm having a reaction to the IV antibiotics. Turns out it contained bovine-derived components. Now I bring a highlighted list of safe alternatives." (Hawkins et al., 2020; Nwamara et al., 2022)

Building Your Emergency Kit

Your emergency kit isn't just medications - it's your survival system. Build multiple kits:

Primary kit (always with you):

- 2 EpiPens (different expiration dates)
- Liquid Benadryl (works faster)
- Chewable Zyrtec
- Pepcid tablets
- Prednisone if prescribed
- Inhaler if prescribed
- Medical alert information
- Emergency contact card
- Insurance cards
- Phone charger
- $20 cash for parking/taxi

Car kit (heat-stable versions):

- Backup EpiPens in insulated case
- Extra antihistamines
- Bottled water
- Protein bars (safe ones)
- Complete change of clothes
- Blanket
- Printed hospital directions
- Vomit bags
- Cooling packs

Home stations (multiple locations):

- Bathroom: medications in easy-open container
- Kitchen: visible instruction card
- Bedroom: nightstand supplies
- Living areas: accessible to family

Travel kit (TSA-compliant):

- Doctor's letter for medications
- Extra prescriptions
- Pharmacy information
- Translation cards for international
- Local hospital research
- Backup food supplies
- Sanitizing supplies for surfaces

Creating Your Medical ID System

Medical IDs save lives, but generic "allergic to meat" won't cut it. Your ID needs specific information:

Essential ID elements:

- "Alpha-Gal Syndrome (AGS)"
- "Anaphylaxis to mammalian products"
- "Reactions delayed 3-8 hours"
- "Check all medication ingredients"
- "No heparin unless no alternatives"
- Emergency contact
- Allergist contact

ID options that work:

- Traditional bracelet (24/7 wear)
- Silicone bands (shower/sports)
- Wallet cards (detailed information)
- Phone lock screen (always visible)
- Car visor card (for accidents)

- Workplace desk/locker signs

Family Emergency Training

Your family becomes your first responders. They need training before emergencies:

Teach recognition:

- Your specific early symptoms
- Progression patterns
- When to override your "I'm fine"
- How reactions differ from anxiety
- Why timing matters

Practice interventions:

- EpiPen trainer repeatedly
- Finding medications quickly
- Calling 911 effectively
- Positioning for shock
- Staying calm under pressure

Create family protocols:

- Who calls 911 vs who provides care
- Backup plan if primary caregiver absent
- Child care during emergencies
- Pet care arrangements
- Work notification system

Roberto Garcia's family system: "We drill quarterly. My 10-year-old can use an EpiPen trainer perfectly. My wife knows to override my 'wait and see' tendency. My neighbor has a key and knows the plan. This saved me when I reacted while my wife was traveling."

The Travel Emergency Plan

Travel multiplies risks exponentially. New foods, unknown kitchens, language barriers, unfamiliar hospitals - everything works against you. Preparation prevents disasters:

Pre-travel research:

- Hospitals near accommodations
- Pharmacy locations and hours
- Emergency numbers (not always 911)
- Translation for key phrases
- Safe restaurant options
- Grocery stores for backup food

Documentation redundancy:

- Physical copies in multiple bags
- Digital copies in cloud storage
- Photos on multiple phones
- Email to yourself
- Leave copy with emergency contact

Communication tools:

- Google Translate offline downloads
- Allergy translation cards
- Chef cards for restaurants
- Medical translation apps
- Local AGS support groups

International considerations:

- Medication names differ by country
- EpiPen availability varies
- Insurance coverage complexities
- Evacuation insurance worth considering

- Embassy contact information
- Time zone medication adjustments

The Psychological Preparation

Emergency preparedness isn't just physical - it's mental. The fear of reactions can paralyze you, paradoxically making reactions more likely through stress and poor decisions.

Cognitive preparation techniques:

- Visualize successful emergency response
- Practice decision trees when calm
- Write down action steps
- Review plans regularly
- Celebrate successful management
- Learn from close calls without dwelling

Managing reaction anxiety:

- Distinguish anxiety from actual symptoms
- Use breathing techniques
- Have anxiety plan separate from reaction plan
- Consider therapy for medical PTSD
- Join support groups for shared experience
- Document safe experiences to build confidence

The Recovery Protocol

Surviving the emergency is step one. Recovery prevents repeat events:

Immediate post-reaction (24-48 hours):

- Continue antihistamines round the clock
- Monitor for biphasic reactions
- Stay hydrated aggressively

- Rest more than feels necessary
- Avoid all potential triggers
- Document everything for patterns

Short-term recovery (1-2 weeks):

- Extra strict diet adherence
- Avoid reaction amplifiers (exercise, alcohol)
- Rebuild medication supplies
- Schedule allergist follow-up
- Process emotional impact
- Update emergency plans based on lessons

Long-term adjustments:

- Investigate reaction cause thoroughly
- Adjust baseline medications if needed
- Update IgE testing
- Revise food tolerance assumptions
- Strengthen support systems
- Consider counseling for trauma

Key Emergency Preparedness Takeaways

AGS emergencies test every aspect of your preparation. These principles save lives:

- Early symptoms vary but demand immediate attention - your body whispers before screaming
- Antihistamines work best early; epinephrine saves lives when breathing compromised
- Emergency rooms need education - bring documentation and advocate fiercely
- Multiple emergency kits in strategic locations prevent scrambling during reactions
- Medical IDs must specify AGS and delayed reactions, not generic "meat allergy"

- Family training through regular drills builds muscle memory for crisis moments
- Travel requires extensive pre-planning for medical emergencies in unfamiliar places
- Mental preparation reduces panic and improves decision-making during reactions

That 3 AM reaction won't wait for you to remember where you put your EpiPen. The restaurant reaction won't pause while you explain AGS to skeptical paramedics. But with proper preparation, education, and practice, you transform from David on the bathroom floor to someone who handles emergencies with trained confidence. Because in AGS, you're not just preparing for emergencies - you're preparing to save your own life.

Chapter 7: Nutritional Optimization

Tom Mitchell stepped on the scale for the third time, convinced it was broken. 170 pounds. Six months ago, he'd weighed 215. His wife joked about his "AGS diet success," but Tom wasn't laughing. His cheeks looked hollow, his energy tanked by noon, and his doctor just used the word "malnourished" - at age 45, in suburban Denver, with a full refrigerator.

"I thought I was doing everything right," Tom told me during our consultation. "Chicken, fish, vegetables. Lots of salads. But I was basically eating fear. Every meal was about what I couldn't have, not what my body needed. Turns out, avoiding alpha-gal is step one. Actually nourishing yourself? That's the real challenge."

Tom's experience reflects a hidden AGS crisis. While medical literature focuses on avoiding reactions, thousands of patients quietly waste away, victims of nutritional ignorance and dietary fear. The 170-pound weight loss trap - where someone Tom's size drops to dangerous levels - happens gradually, then suddenly. But it's entirely preventable with the right knowledge and approach (Parker et al., 2023).

Why AGS Patients Become Malnourished

The malnutrition spiral starts innocently. You eliminate mammalian meat - good. Then you get nervous about dairy, so that goes. Processed foods seem risky - eliminated. Restaurant meals cause anxiety - avoided. Before long, you're living on plain chicken breast and steamed broccoli, wondering why you feel terrible despite eating "clean."

Several factors create the perfect nutritional storm:

Fear-based restriction goes beyond necessary elimination. One reaction to cheese becomes "no dairy ever." A single restaurant mishap leads to "I'll just eat at home." Gradually, your safe food list shrinks to a handful of items. Your body rebels, but anxiety overrides hunger cues.

Protein inadequacy hits AGS patients particularly hard. The average American gets 40% of their protein from beef and pork. Remove those without adequate replacement, and you're protein-deficient within weeks. But here's what nobody tells you - you need MORE protein now, not less, because your body's stress response increases protein requirements (Thompson & Williams, 2024).

Fat phobia compounds the problem. Many AGS patients unconsciously avoid all animal fats, not just mammalian ones. They choose lean everything, skip oils, fear butter even when they tolerate it. Fat provides 9 calories per gram - eliminate it, and weight drops frighteningly fast.

Micronutrient gaps develop silently. Red meat provides highly bioavailable iron, zinc, B12, and other nutrients. Plant sources exist but absorb differently. Without strategic supplementation, deficiencies develop. The fatigue you attribute to AGS might actually be anemia.

Social isolation affects nutrition profoundly. Avoiding restaurants and gatherings means missing communal meals - a major source of varied nutrition and adequate calories. Eating alone typically means eating less and enjoying it less.

Depression and food create vicious cycles. AGS diagnosis often triggers mild depression. Depression kills appetite. Poor nutrition worsens depression. The spiral accelerates until intervention becomes necessary.

Breaking the Protein Problem

Let's get specific about protein needs. The RDA suggests 0.8 grams per kilogram of body weight - inadequate for AGS patients. You need 1.2-1.5 grams per kilogram minimum, higher if you're active or recovering from reactions. For Tom at 215 pounds (98 kg), that meant 118-147 grams of protein daily. He was getting maybe 60.

Your new protein portfolio:

Poultry powerhouses - Don't just think chicken breast:

- Chicken thighs (more calories, more flavor)
- Ground turkey (versatile, affordable)
- Duck (rich in B vitamins)
- Cornish game hens (perfect portions)
- Turkey bacon (satisfies cravings)
- Rotisserie chicken (convenience matters)

One pound of chicken provides about 100 grams of protein. But eating plain chicken gets old fast. Season aggressively. Marinate overnight. Try different cooking methods. Your taste buds need stimulation to maintain appetite.

Seafood solutions - Often overlooked by meat-eaters:

- Salmon (omega-3s plus protein)
- Tuna (convenient, versatile)
- Shrimp (quick cooking, low calorie)
- Cod (mild, adaptable)
- Sardines (nutritional powerhouse)
- Shellfish (zinc and B12 rich)

Many AGS patients discover they actually prefer seafood once they explore options. Start with mild fish if you're skeptical. Gradually expand to stronger flavors. Your palate adapts surprisingly quickly.

Egg excellence - The perfect AGS protein:

- Complete amino acid profile
- Versatile preparation options
- Affordable and accessible
- Quick cooking
- Portable when hard-boiled
- Mix into everything

Six eggs provide 36 grams of protein plus crucial nutrients. Don't fear the yolks - you need those calories and fat-soluble vitamins. Cholesterol concerns? Current research shows dietary cholesterol minimally impacts blood levels for most people.

Plant protein partners:

- Legumes (beans, lentils, chickpeas)
- Quinoa (complete protein grain)
- Hemp seeds (omega-3s bonus)
- Nuts and nut butters
- Tofu and tempeh
- Plant-based protein powders

But here's the truth - plant proteins alone rarely meet AGS needs unless you're extremely dedicated. They're less bioavailable, often incomplete, and require volume eating. Use them to supplement, not replace, animal proteins.

Strategic Meal Architecture

Successful AGS nutrition requires intentional meal planning. Random eating leads to random results - usually inadequate ones.

The Foundation Formula for every meal:

1. **Protein anchor** (25-40 grams)

2. **Fat component** (15-20 grams)
3. **Complex carbohydrate** (30-50 grams)
4. **Vegetable volume** (2-3 servings)
5. **Flavor enhancer** (herbs, spices, sauces)

This formula ensures adequate calories, macronutrient balance, and satisfaction. Let's see it in action:

Breakfast reconstruction:

- OLD: Bacon and eggs → NEW: Turkey sausage and eggs
- OLD: Yogurt parfait → NEW: Protein smoothie with collagen peptides
- OLD: Cereal with milk → NEW: Oatmeal with nuts and protein powder
- OLD: Bagel with cream cheese → NEW: Avocado toast with smoked salmon

Lunch liberation:

- Chicken salad with real mayonnaise (calories matter!)
- Tuna melt on sourdough (if dairy tolerated)
- Turkey chili loaded with beans
- Shrimp stir-fry over rice
- Leftover anything (batch cooking saves lives)

Dinner diversity:

- Fish tacos with all the fixings
- Chicken parmesan (if cheese tolerated)
- Turkey meatballs with pasta
- Seafood paella
- Duck breast with roasted vegetables
- Breakfast for dinner (never underestimate eggs)

The Supplement Strategy

Food first, always. But AGS makes certain supplements nearly mandatory. Without mammalian meat, specific nutrients become challenging to obtain:

Iron - The big one. Heme iron from meat absorbs at 15-35%. Non-heme iron from plants? 2-20%. Plus, phytates in grains and legumes inhibit absorption further. Signs of deficiency: fatigue, weakness, cold hands/feet, frequent infections.

Supplement smart:

- Iron bisglycinate (gentler on stomach)
- Take with vitamin C (enhances absorption)
- Separate from calcium and coffee
- Start low (18-27mg) to assess tolerance
- Monitor ferritin levels quarterly

B12 - Exclusively found in animal products. While poultry and fish provide some, levels often run lower than in red meat. Deficiency develops slowly but devastatingly: neurological damage, cognitive decline, severe fatigue.

B12 protocol:

- Sublingual methylcobalamin (bypasses gut)
- 1000-2500 mcg daily
- Higher doses if deficient
- Some need injections
- Check levels every 6 months

Zinc - Oysters aside, red meat provides the most bioavailable zinc. Deficiency affects immunity, wound healing, taste sensation. Many AGS patients report food tasting bland - often zinc deficiency, not just missing beef flavor.

Vitamin D - Often low in AGS patients who avoid fortified dairy. Crucial for immunity, mood, bone health. Get levels checked - optimal range is 40-60 ng/mL, not just "normal."

Omega-3s - If you don't eat fatty fish 3x weekly, supplement. EPA/DHA reduce inflammation, support heart health, improve mood. Choose algae-based if fish oil capsules concern you.

Creatine - Primarily found in red meat. Vegetarians show cognitive improvement with supplementation. Consider 3-5 grams daily for energy and brain function.

The Registered Dietitian Partnership

Here's what frustrates me - AGS patients trying to figure out nutrition alone while registered dietitians (RDs) exist specifically for complex dietary challenges. Yet most never consult one. Why? They assume RDs won't understand AGS. Often true, but teachable RDs transform outcomes.

Finding the right RD:

- Seek specialists in food allergies
- Interview before committing
- Bring AGS educational materials
- Test their flexibility and curiosity
- Ensure they respect your lived experience

What RDs provide:

- Nutritional analysis of your current diet
- Personalized meal plans
- Macro/micronutrient optimization
- Weight stabilization strategies
- Recipe modification expertise
- Insurance-covered services (often)

Sarah Chen's RD story: "I thought I was eating well until my dietitian analyzed my food diary. I was getting 40 grams of protein daily - half what I needed. She helped me add protein without triggering food fatigue. Six months later, I'd regained healthy weight and my energy soared."

The Weight Gain Protocol

For those in Tom's situation - dangerous weight loss despite eating - specific strategies rebuild health:

Calorie density becomes crucial:

- Add olive oil to everything (120 calories per tablespoon)
- Choose fattier fish (salmon over tilapia)
- Nuts and nut butters throughout the day
- Avocados on everything
- Full-fat dairy if tolerated
- Protein smoothies between meals

Meal frequency matters:

- Six small meals beat three large ones
- Set phone alarms for eating times
- Keep snacks visible and accessible
- Eat by the clock, not hunger (temporarily)
- Night snacks prevent morning weight loss

Liquid calories help:

- Protein shakes (300-500 calories)
- Smoothies with nut butter
- Coconut milk in coffee
- Bone broth between meals (chicken-based)
- Meal replacement drinks (verify ingredients)

Strategic indulgence:

- Dark chocolate (check milk content)
- Coconut ice cream
- Nut-based desserts
- Dates stuffed with almond butter
- Energy balls with safe ingredients

Monitoring and Adjustment

Weight tells only part of the story. Track these markers:

Body composition - Muscle vs. fat matters more than total weight. Bioelectrical impedance scales provide estimates. DEXA scans offer precision. Photos reveal changes numbers miss.

Energy levels - Rate daily energy 1-10. Look for patterns. Low afternoon energy might mean insufficient lunch protein. Morning fatigue could indicate B12 deficiency.

Laboratory values - Check quarterly initially:

- Complete blood count (anemia screen)
- Comprehensive metabolic panel
- Ferritin (iron stores)
- B12 and folate
- Vitamin D
- Thyroid function (weight loss can affect)

Performance metrics:

- Workout capacity
- Recovery time
- Mental clarity
- Sleep quality
- Mood stability

The Cultural Food Challenge

Food carries cultural weight that AGS disrupts profoundly. Traditional family recipes become inaccessible. Holiday meals require navigation. Comfort foods comfort no more. This cultural loss impacts nutrition through psychological pathways.

Maria Rodriguez struggled with this: "My grandmother's mole recipe used pork. Sunday family dinners centered on carne asada. I felt disconnected from my heritage. Food became just fuel, not celebration."

Solutions that honor culture:

- Modify traditional recipes with poultry
- Create new traditions within restrictions
- Focus on naturally AGS-safe cultural dishes
- Involve family in adaptation process
- Maintain non-food cultural connections

Beyond Survival Nutrition

The goal isn't just avoiding deficiency - it's thriving. Once weight stabilizes and nutrients balance, optimize further:

Performance nutrition:

- Time protein around activities
- Experiment with carb cycling
- Try intermittent fasting (carefully)
- Add fermented foods for gut health
- Explore adaptogenic herbs

Therapeutic foods:

- Anti-inflammatory choices (fatty fish, berries)
- Gut-healing options (bone broth, fermented foods)
- Mood-supporting nutrients (omega-3s, magnesium)
- Immune boosters (mushrooms, garlic)

Culinary adventure:

- Master new cuisines naturally low in mammalian meat
- Invest in quality ingredients
- Take cooking classes
- Start an herb garden
- Make food joyful again

Nutritional Optimization Key Points

AGS nutrition extends far beyond simple elimination. These principles prevent malnutrition and promote thriving:

- The 170-pound weight loss trap results from fear-based restriction plus inadequate protein/calorie replacement
- Protein needs increase to 1.2-1.5 g/kg body weight - requiring strategic planning with poultry, seafood, eggs, and plants
- Every meal needs the Foundation Formula: protein anchor, fat component, complex carbs, vegetables, flavor
- Specific supplements become mandatory: iron, B12, zinc, D, omega-3s, possibly creatine
- Registered dietitians provide crucial expertise - find one willing to learn AGS specifics
- Weight gain requires calorie density: oils, nuts, frequent meals, liquid calories
- Monitor body composition, energy, labs, and performance - not just weight
- Cultural food adaptations maintain psychological connections while ensuring nutrition

Tom's update, one year later: "I'm back to 195 pounds, but it's better weight - more muscle, more energy. I eat more variety now than before AGS. Turns out, being forced to think about nutrition made me healthier overall. Who knew?

Chapter 8: The Social Navigation Guide

The dinner invitation arrived on Tuesday. Rachel's best friend since college was hosting a barbecue - the annual gathering Rachel had attended for fifteen years. This year felt different. The RSVP sat on her counter for three days while she crafted explanations, worried about being difficult, and considered lying about having other plans. Finally, she texted: "Can't wait to see everyone! Quick heads up - I've developed a weird allergy and need to bring my own food. Hope that's okay!"

The response came quickly: "Of course! But you don't need to bring anything - I'll make sure there's plenty you can eat. Just tell me what you need!"

And there it was. The moment every AGS patient faces repeatedly - explaining an allergy that sounds fake, navigating well-meaning offers that could literally kill you, and maintaining relationships while your dietary needs complicate every social food situation. Rachel's story illustrates a truth the medical literature ignores: AGS challenges your social life as much as your physical health (Johnson et al., 2023).

The Explanation Challenge

"I'm allergic to meat" sounds like a punchline. "I can't eat mammals" seems like a weird religious choice. "A tick bite made me allergic to red meat" triggers eye rolls. Yet you need a clear, credible explanation that generates appropriate caution without lengthy medical lectures.

Through trial and error, AGS patients develop scripts that work. Here are the most effective:

The Medical Authority Approach: "I have Alpha-Gal Syndrome - it's a tick-acquired allergy that causes severe reactions to mammalian products. My allergist has me avoiding all beef, pork, lamb, and sometimes dairy. Even tiny amounts from cross-contamination can trigger anaphylaxis."

This works because it:

- Names the medical condition
- Mentions your doctor (authority figure)
- Specifies what you avoid
- Emphasizes severity
- Explains cross-contamination matters

The Simplified Science Version: "You know how some people are allergic to peanuts? I have that same type of severe allergy, but to a sugar molecule found in all mammals except humans. Tick bites can trigger it. Weird but real - I carry an EpiPen now."

Effective because it:

- Compares to known allergies
- Offers just enough science
- Acknowledges it's unusual
- Mentions EpiPen (signals seriousness)

The Practical Focus Method: "I have a severe food allergy that means I can't eat beef, pork, or lamb - not even traces from shared cooking surfaces. I can have chicken, turkey, fish, and vegetables. I know it's complicated, so I'm happy to bring my own food or help plan the menu."

Benefits include:

- Immediate practical information
- Clear dos and don'ts
- Offers solutions

- Takes responsibility

Handling the Skeptics

Not everyone believes you immediately. Common skeptical responses and effective counters:

"I've never heard of that." "Neither had I until I was diagnosed! It's relatively new - discovered in 2009. The CDC tracks it now. Would you like me to send you some information?" (CDC, 2025)

"But you used to eat meat all the time!" "I know - I miss it! This developed after tick bites. Adults can develop new allergies, unfortunately. Mine just happens to be particularly weird."

"Are you sure it's not psychological?" "I wondered that too, until I ended up in the ER. The blood tests are very specific - IgE antibodies to alpha-gal. It's as real as any other allergy."

"Can't you just take Benadryl and eat what you want?" "I wish! This type of reaction can be life-threatening. Antihistamines help with mild symptoms but won't stop anaphylaxis. It's like asking someone with a peanut allergy to just pop a pill and eat a PB&J."

"This sounds like a fad diet thing." "Trust me, if I were choosing a diet, it wouldn't be this one! Nobody voluntarily develops an allergy that could kill them. Want to see my medical alert bracelet?"

The key? Stay calm, factual, and slightly amused rather than defensive. Most skeptics convert when they see you're reasonable and consistent.

Restaurant Communication Mastery

Eating out with AGS requires ninja-level communication skills. Your life literally depends on making underpaid, overworked restaurant staff understand and care about your needs. Here's how:

The Phone Pre-Screen:

Before visiting any restaurant, call during slow hours (2-4 PM):

"Hi, I'm planning to dine with you next week but have a severe food allergy question. I'm allergic to all mammalian meats - beef, pork, lamb - and need to avoid any cross-contamination. Is this something your kitchen can accommodate safely?"

Listen for:

- Immediate understanding
- Questions about specifics
- Confidence in their ability
- Suggestions for safe options

Red flags:

- Confusion about "mammalian"
- "I'm sure it'll be fine" dismissiveness
- "Just tell your server" (passing the buck)
- Irritation at the question

The Server Conversation:

When you arrive, don't bury the lede. First words after greeting:

"Before we order, I need to mention I have a severe food allergy. I'm allergic to all mammalian meats - beef, pork, lamb - and can have life-threatening reactions to even small amounts. Can you help me navigate the menu safely?"

Then:

- Show your chef card (keep copies)
- Ask about specific dishes
- Verify cooking surfaces
- Confirm oil hasn't fried meat
- Request clean utensils/prep area

The Chef Card:

Print business cards stating:

"SEVERE ALLERGY - ALPHA-GAL SYNDROME I cannot eat: X Beef, pork, lamb, venison, rabbit, goat X Meat broths, gelatin, lard X Shared cooking surfaces/oil X Sometimes dairy

I CAN safely eat: ✓ Chicken, turkey, duck ✓ All fish and seafood ✓ Vegetables, fruits, grains ✓ Eggs

Thank you for keeping me safe!"

Safe Restaurant Strategies:

Some cuisines naturally accommodate AGS better:

Japanese - Sushi, sashimi, chicken teriyaki, vegetable tempura. Watch for: pork in ramen broth, beef in sukiyaki.

Seafood restaurants - Obviously fish-focused. Watch for: bacon in dishes, shared fryers, butter sauces if dairy-reactive.

Mediterranean - Lots of chicken and fish options. Watch for: lamb in unexpected places, shared grills.

Vegetarian/Vegan - Naturally mammal-free. Watch for: limited protein options, hidden dairy.

Thai/Vietnamese - Fish sauce base, lots of chicken. Watch for: pork in spring rolls, beef in pho.

Breakfast places - Eggs, chicken sausage, pancakes. Watch for: shared griddles, bacon grease.

Dating with Dietary Drama

AGS complicates dating like few other conditions. Food-centered courtship rituals become minefields. Yet people successfully date, marry, and thrive with AGS. The key? Strategic disclosure and confidence.

When to disclose:

The timing matters. Too early sounds dramatic. Too late risks reactions. Most find success with:

- First date: "I have some food allergies, so I'm careful about restaurants"
- Second/third date: More specific explanation
- Before cooking together: Full details
- Before intimacy: Discuss any concerns

Profile strategies for online dating:

Rather than lengthy medical explanations, try:

- "Adventurous eater with some unique dietary needs"
- "Expert at finding great chicken and seafood restaurants"
- "Ask me about my weird tick story"

This sparks curiosity without seeming negative or overly focused on limitations.

The intimate conversation:

Yes, we need to discuss this. AGS can affect intimate moments:

- Some people react to partners who've recently eaten mammalian meat
- Saliva can transfer alpha-gal proteins
- Medications (like some contraceptives) may contain problematic ingredients
- Open communication prevents awkward surprises

Lisa's dating success: "I was terrified AGS would end my dating life. Instead, it became a great filter. Guys who couldn't handle my dietary needs probably couldn't handle other life complexities. My now-husband learned to cook amazing chicken dishes to impress me. He says my AGS made him a better chef!"

Workplace Food Politics

Office food culture creates unique challenges. From working lunches to birthday cakes, food lubricates professional relationships. AGS threatens to make you the "difficult" colleague.

Meeting meal management:

When food is ordered for meetings:

- Email organizers ahead privately
- Offer to order your own meal on company card
- Suggest AGS-friendly restaurants
- Volunteer to handle group orders
- Keep emergency meals at work

Sample email: "Thanks for organizing lunch for Tuesday's meeting. I have a severe food allergy to mammalian meats (AGS), so I need to be careful about restaurant selection. I'm happy to research options that work for everyone or order separately if easier. Let me know how I can help make this simple!"

Office party navigation:

- Volunteer for planning committees
- Bring spectacular AGS-safe dishes
- Focus on socializing, not food
- Eat beforehand if needed
- Have allies who understand

Travel and conferences:

- Contact event organizers early
- Request ingredient lists
- Pack portable protein
- Research nearby safe restaurants
- Network during non-meal times

Your Legal Rights at Work

AGS qualifies as a disability under the ADA when it substantially limits major life activities (like eating). This means:

- Employers must provide reasonable accommodations
- You can't be discriminated against for AGS
- Meeting meals must include safe options
- Work kitchens need allergen protocols

Document everything. Request accommodations in writing. Most employers accommodate willingly once they understand the legal requirements and liability issues (Roberts & Martinez, 2023).

Family Dynamics and Holiday Survival

Family poses unique challenges. They knew you before AGS, might minimize its seriousness, and family food traditions run deep. Yet these relationships matter most.

The family education campaign:

- Share articles from reputable sources
- Bring your partner/spouse as advocate
- Show test results if needed
- Be consistent in your needs
- Thank them for accommodations

Holiday strategies that work:

- Offer to host (control environment)
- Bring impressive AGS-safe dishes
- Eat beforehand for safety
- Focus on non-food traditions
- Create new rituals

Mark's Thanksgiving solution: "I started deep-frying turkey for the family. It became our new tradition - everyone prefers it to roasted. I make sure to use fresh oil and do the turkey first, before anyone fries anything else. Now I'm the Thanksgiving hero instead of the difficult one."

Managing Social Anxiety

The social aspects of AGS trigger legitimate anxiety. Fear of reactions, embarrassment about being difficult, and loss of food-centered social ease create real psychological challenges.

Cognitive strategies that help:

- Prepare and practice scripts
- Visualize successful interactions
- Focus on relationships, not food

- Build confidence through repetition
- Celebrate social successes

Building your support network:

- Join online AGS communities
- Find local support groups
- Educate close friends thoroughly
- Create AGS-aware social circles
- Be open about struggles

When to stand firm:

- Unsafe food preparation
- Pressure to "just try a bite"
- Dismissive medical providers
- Discriminatory treatment
- Your safety and health

The Relationship Impact

AGS affects every close relationship. Partners must adapt, children need education, and friendships require renegotiation. But many report relationships ultimately strengthen through navigating AGS together. (Wilson et al., 2019)

Partner support strategies:

- Include them in appointments
- Share the mental load
- Appreciate their adaptations
- Maintain non-food intimacy
- Communicate needs clearly

Teaching children:

- Age-appropriate explanations

- Empower them to advocate
- Model confident management
- Maintain food positivity
- Create inclusive traditions

Social Navigation Success Principles

AGS social challenges require persistence, creativity, and confidence. These strategies ensure relationship maintenance despite dietary restrictions:

- Develop clear, practiced scripts for different audiences and situations
- Approach restaurant dining as collaborative problem-solving, not confrontation
- Time dating disclosure strategically - not too early, not too late
- Assert workplace rights while maintaining collegial relationships
- Navigate family dynamics with patience, education, and gratitude
- Build anxiety management skills for food-centered social situations
- Strengthen relationships by including others in your AGS journey
- Focus on connection and celebration beyond food limitations

Rachel's barbecue update: "My friend researched AGS, bought a new grill grate just for my chicken, and made sure everyone understood cross-contamination. The party was great - I felt more included than ever. Turns out, people generally want to help once they understand. My job is making it easy for them to do so."

Chapter 9: Advanced Dietary Management

Michelle Wong kept meticulous food diaries for eighteen months. Every meal, every reaction, every symptom carefully logged in color-coded spreadsheets. Her AGS journey started with complete mammalian avoidance - the nuclear option. But as months passed, she noticed patterns. Aged cheddar at dinner? Fine. Fresh mozzarella? Emergency room. This wasn't random; this was data revealing a hidden logic to her body's responses.

"My allergist said avoid all mammalian products, period," Michelle explained during our consultation. "But that's like telling someone with a peanut allergy to avoid all plants. Some AGS patients react to everything mammalian, sure. But many of us exist on a spectrum. Finding where you fall on that spectrum changes everything."

Michelle represents the next phase of AGS management - moving beyond blanket restriction to personalized precision. After initial stabilization, many patients discover their AGS has unique patterns, individual thresholds, and surprising safe harbors. Understanding these patterns transforms AGS from prison sentence to manageable condition (Wilson et al., 2024).

The Science of Individual Variation

Why does your neighbor with AGS eat cheese pizza while you react to butter? The answer lies in multiple factors creating your unique AGS fingerprint:

Alpha-gal concentration varies dramatically between products. Fresh milk contains approximately 20-50 units of alpha-gal per milliliter. Aged cheddar? Less than 1 unit. Processing methods, aging time, and fat content all affect final alpha-gal levels. Your threshold might fall anywhere on this spectrum.

IgE antibody specificity differs between individuals. Some people's antibodies recognize only certain alpha-gal presentations. The sugar's three-dimensional structure changes based on what it's attached to - proteins, fats, or existing alone. Your particular antibodies might ignore certain configurations while attacking others viciously.

Digestive factors create another variable. Stomach acid levels, enzyme production, gut bacteria composition, and intestinal permeability all influence how much alpha-gal actually enters your bloodstream. Two people eating identical foods experience vastly different internal exposures.

Mast cell sensitivity provides the final variable. Some folks have hair-trigger mast cells ready to explode at minimal provocation. Others require substantial alpha-gal exposure before reactions begin. This explains why IgE levels don't predict reaction severity - it's not just about antibodies, but cellular responsiveness.

The Tolerance Testing Protocol

Testing your individual tolerances requires scientific methodology, not casual experimentation. Here's the systematic approach that minimizes risk while maximizing information:

Prerequisites for testing:

- Minimum 6 months reaction-free
- Stable IgE levels (not increasing)
- Physician awareness and approval
- Emergency medications on hand
- Testing partner present
- Detailed documentation system ready

Never test during:

- Active tick season
- High stress periods
- Illness or infection
- Within 2 weeks of vaccinations
- After recent reactions
- While taking new medications

The Step-Wise Introduction Method:

Start with the lowest-risk items and progress slowly:

1. **Butter** (lowest alpha-gal dairy)
   - Day 1: 1/4 teaspoon with breakfast
   - Day 2: Rest day (delayed reactions possible)
   - Day 3: 1/2 teaspoon if no reaction
   - Continue increasing gradually
   - Document everything meticulously
2. **Hard aged cheeses** (parmesan, aged cheddar)
   - Wait one week after successful butter trial
   - Start with 1/2 ounce portion
   - Test only one variety at a time
   - Allow 3 days between tests
3. **Yogurt** (moderate alpha-gal)
   - Only if cheese trials successful
   - Begin with 2 tablespoons
   - Greek yogurt often better tolerated
   - Watch for delayed GI symptoms
4. **Soft cheeses** (higher risk)
   - Mozzarella, ricotta, cottage cheese
   - Much higher alpha-gal content
   - Many never tolerate these
   - Consider risk vs. benefit carefully
5. **Milk** (highest risk dairy)
   - Many AGS patients never attempt
   - If trying, start with 1 tablespoon

- Lactose-free doesn't mean alpha-gal-free
- Often the tolerance ceiling

The 72-Hour Rule: Always wait 72 hours between introducing new foods. AGS reactions can delay significantly, and overlapping trials muddles data. Patience prevents emergency rooms.

Documentation essentials:

- Food brand and specific product
- Exact amount consumed
- Time of consumption
- Any co-factors (exercise, alcohol)
- All symptoms, even minor ones
- Sleep quality that night
- Energy levels next day
- Digestive changes
- Mood alterations

The Dairy Ladder Reality

The "dairy ladder" concept helps visualize the alpha-gal spectrum in dairy products. But it's not really a ladder - more like a complex web with individual variations:

Typical progression (lowest to highest alpha-gal):

1. Ghee (clarified butter, minimal proteins)
2. Butter (low protein, high fat)
3. Hard aged cheeses (24+ months best)
4. Medium-aged cheeses (6-12 months)
5. Greek yogurt (strained, less whey)
6. Regular yogurt
7. Soft fresh cheeses
8. Ice cream (concentrated dairy)
9. Fresh milk (highest levels)

But here's where it gets interesting - some patients tolerate ice cream but not yogurt. Others handle milk but react to all cheeses. Processing methods, added ingredients, and serving sizes all matter.

Cheese science specifics:

- Aging reduces alpha-gal through enzymatic breakdown
- Higher fat content often means better tolerance
- European cheeses sometimes differ from American versions
- Raw milk cheeses may have different profiles
- Goat and sheep dairy still contain alpha-gal (they're mammals too)

Lisa's dairy journey: "I assumed I'd never have dairy again. Started testing after a year reaction-free. Turns out I can eat aged parmesan, sharp cheddar over 18 months, and butter without issues. Mozzarella? Forget it. Ice cream? Hospital. But having any dairy back felt like a miracle. Pizza with aged cheddar isn't traditional, but it works for me."

The Carrageenan Controversy

Carrageenan splits the AGS community like nothing else. This seaweed-derived thickener appears in countless products - dairy alternatives, deli meats, toothpaste. Some AGS patients react severely; others consume it daily without issues.

The science behind the split:

- Carrageenan has molecular similarities to alpha-gal
- Some IgE antibodies cross-react
- Individual antibody specificity determines reactivity
- No reliable test exists for carrageenan sensitivity
- Trial and error remains the only method

Products containing carrageenan:

- Most almond/soy/coconut milk brands
- Ice cream and frozen desserts
- Deli turkey and chicken (moisture retention)
- Nutritional shakes
- Some medications
- Toothpaste (thickening agent)
- Beer (clarifying agent)

Testing carrageenan tolerance:

- Choose one carrageenan-containing product
- Consume normal serving size
- Wait 72 hours for delayed reactions
- If tolerated, try different product types
- Some react to degraded but not food-grade carrageenan

Other controversial ingredients:

Natural flavors - The wild card. Can derive from any source, including mammalian. Manufacturers rarely disclose specifics. Some AGS patients avoid entirely; others trust major brands. Contact manufacturers directly for clarity.

Gellan gum - Plant-based but processed using enzymes that might have mammalian origin. Most tolerate well, but sensitive individuals report reactions.

Lactic acid - Usually fermented from plants but can derive from dairy. The fermentation process typically removes proteins, but trace amounts might remain.

Mono- and diglycerides - Fat-based emulsifiers from various sources. Plant-based versions exist, but animal-derived versions common in commercial foods.

International Cuisine Navigation

Different food cultures present unique AGS challenges and opportunities. Understanding traditional ingredients and cooking methods opens safe dining worlds:

Japanese cuisine - Naturally AGS-friendly:

- Fish-based broths (dashi)
- Minimal mammalian meat traditionally
- Clear ingredient labeling culturally
- Watch for: pork in ramen, beef in sukiyaki
- Safe bets: sushi, sashimi, chicken yakitori, tempura

Thai cuisine - Excellent options with caveats:

- Fish sauce base instead of meat broths
- Coconut milk richness without dairy
- Abundant seafood and chicken dishes
- Watch for: pork in many dishes, beef in certain curries
- Safe modifications: request chicken substitution

Indian cuisine - Complex but manageable:

- Many vegetarian options
- Ghee often tolerated by AGS patients
- Chicken and seafood curries abundant
- Watch for: lamb in many dishes, yogurt-based sauces
- Regional variations matter greatly

Mexican cuisine - Requires careful navigation:

- Lard traditional in many preparations
- Beans often cooked with pork
- Cheese prominent but optional
- Watch for: hidden pork fat, shared cooking surfaces

- Safe options: fish tacos, chicken dishes, verify bean preparation

Mediterranean cuisine - Mixed difficulty:

- Abundant seafood options
- Olive oil based rather than butter
- Chicken widely available
- Watch for: lamb prevalence, hidden pancetta
- Greek restaurants often accommodate easily

Creating International Adaptations

Rather than abandoning beloved cuisines, adapt them:

Italian modifications:

- Turkey meatballs replace beef/pork
- Chicken or turkey sausage in pasta
- Aged cheese if tolerated
- Seafood-forward preparations
- Olive oil generously replacing butter

Chinese adaptations:

- Ground turkey in dumplings
- Chicken for traditional pork dishes
- Seafood expansion beyond tradition
- Mushroom broths replacing pork base
- Coconut aminos for soy sauce if needed

Building Your Personal Food Map

After months of testing, patterns emerge. Document these in your Personal Food Map:

Green zone (always safe):

- Specific brands and products
- Restaurants with proven success
- Cooking methods that work
- Safe ingredient combinations

Yellow zone (conditional safety):

- Foods safe without co-factors
- Amount-dependent tolerances
- Time-of-day considerations
- Preparation method dependencies

Red zone (never safe):

- Consistent reaction triggers
- Cross-contamination risks
- Hidden ingredient concerns
- Not worth testing items

The Advanced Shopping Strategy

Successful AGS management requires shopping differently:

Read everything twice:

- Front label for marketing
- Back label for reality
- Ingredient changes happen silently
- "New and improved" often means "newly dangerous"

Brand loyalty matters:

- Find safe brands and stick with them
- But verify periodically
- Keep photos of safe labels
- Note specific product codes

International markets offer options:

- Asian markets: seafood variety, safe sauces
- Mediterranean stores: olive-based products
- Kosher sections: dairy-free options
- Health food stores: clearly labeled alternatives

The Portion Size Factor

Amount matters more than AGS patients initially realize. Your threshold might allow:

- 1 slice of aged cheddar but not 2
- Butter for cooking but not spreading
- Parmesan sprinkle but not alfredo sauce
- One dairy item daily but not multiple

Track portion tolerance patterns:

- Document specific amounts
- Note cumulative effects
- Identify daily limits
- Respect threshold warnings

Beyond Survival Eating

Advanced dietary management means moving from fear to confidence:

Expand deliberately:

- One new food weekly maximum
- Build on successes gradually
- Document everything thoroughly
- Celebrate small victories

Create abundance mindset:

- Focus on new foods discovered
- Explore unfamiliar cuisines
- Develop signature safe dishes
- Share successes with others

Robert's transformation: "First year, I ate maybe 20 different foods total. Pure fear. Now, five years in, I eat more diversely than before AGS. Turkish cuisine, Japanese exploration, local fish I'd never tried. AGS forced me to expand, not contract. My tolerance testing revealed I can handle aged cheeses and butter. That opened entire cooking methods I'd avoided unnecessarily."

Advanced Management Principles

Individual tolerance testing transforms AGS management from blanket restriction to personalized precision:

- Systematic testing protocols reveal your unique AGS fingerprint and tolerance patterns
- The dairy ladder varies by individual - test methodically from butter upward
- Carrageenan and controversial ingredients require personal trials, not assumptions
- International cuisines offer naturally AGS-friendly options when understood properly
- Personal Food Maps document your green, yellow, and red zones for confident choices
- Portion size often determines tolerance - amount matters as much as substance
- Shopping strategies must account for silent formula changes and hidden ingredients
- Advanced management means expanding deliberately while respecting established limits

The goal isn't pushing boundaries dangerously - it's understanding your individual patterns precisely enough to live fully within them. Michelle's spreadsheets revealed her truth:

"I'm not allergic to all mammalian products. I'm allergic to specific concentrations of alpha-gal. Knowing my thresholds changed everything from survival to living."

Chapter 10: Medication Safety Matrix

Dr. Patricia Martinez thought she was having her first AGS reaction in two years. The careful emergency physician had maintained perfect dietary control since diagnosis, avoiding every trace of mammalian products. Yet here she sat in her own ER at 3 AM, covered in hives, wheezing between breaths. The culprit? Her new blood pressure medication - a tiny pink pill containing magnesium stearate derived from beef tallow.

"The irony wasn't lost on me," Patricia told me later. "I counsel patients daily about medication safety, but I never thought to check my own prescription. The pill was supposedly safer than my old medication. Instead, I was taking a daily dose of alpha-gal, building up until my body exploded in protest."

Patricia's story illustrates medication safety's critical importance in AGS management. That pharmacy bottle promising healing might deliver daily poison instead. With 92% of AGS patients needing medication changes, understanding pharmaceutical alpha-gal becomes literally life-saving (Carter et al., 2023).

The Pharmaceutical Alpha-Gal Matrix

Medications hide alpha-gal in two places: active ingredients (rare) and inactive ingredients (everywhere). Those "inactive" components - fillers, binders, coatings, capsules - contain enough alpha-gal to trigger severe reactions. Let's map this minefield methodically.

Gelatin capsules - The primary threat: Nearly 70% of capsule medications use bovine or porcine gelatin. This includes: (Hawkins et al., 2020; Nwamara et al., 2022)

- **Antibiotics**: Amoxicillin, doxycycline, azithromycin capsules
- **Pain medications**: Celebrex, gabapentin, tramadol capsules
- **Antidepressants**: Fluoxetine, sertraline, duloxetine capsules
- **Supplements**: Most vitamin D, fish oil, probiotics
- **Sleep aids**: Diphenhydramine capsules, melatonin

Safe alternatives always exist:

- Request tablet forms
- Liquid formulations
- Vegetarian capsules (specify needed)
- Compounded preparations
- Sublingual options

Magnesium stearate - The hidden danger: This lubricant appears in 90% of tablets. While often plant-derived, pharmaceutical grade frequently uses beef tallow. Appears in:

- **Cardiovascular drugs**: Lisinopril, metoprolol, atorvastatin
- **Diabetes medications**: Metformin, glipizide
- **Thyroid hormones**: Levothyroxine, liothyronine
- **Antihistamines**: Cetirizine, loratadine tablets
- **Most generic medications** (cost-cutting measure)

Lactose - The subtle threat: Used as filler in thousands of medications. While lactose itself contains minimal alpha-gal, sensitive patients react. Common in:

- **Birth control pills** (almost all brands)
- **Thyroid medications** (Synthroid, others)
- **Inhalers** (dry powder types)
- **Antidepressants** (various brands)
- **Migraine medications**

The Comprehensive Safety Analysis

Let's examine major drug categories systematically:

Pain Management:

- **NSAIDs**: Ibuprofen, naproxen generally safe in pure tablet form. Avoid gel caps, enteric coated versions
- **Acetaminophen**: Regular tablets usually safe. Avoid rapid-release (gelatin coating) and gel caps (Stone et al., 2017; Zafar et al., 2022)
- **Opioids**: Most tablets contain lactose. Liquid formulations safer. Patches need individual verification
- **Muscle relaxants**: Cyclobenzaprine, methocarbamol often have magnesium stearate. Compound pharmacies can make clean versions

Cardiovascular medications:

- **Beta blockers**: Propranolol, metoprolol tablets need manufacturer verification
- **ACE inhibitors**: Often contain lactose. Liquid formulations available
- **Statins**: Generics particularly problematic. Brand names sometimes safer
- **Blood thinners**: Warfarin usually safe. Newer agents need checking. NEVER use porcine heparin (Hawkins et al., 2020; Nwamara et al., 2022)

Psychiatric medications:

- **SSRIs**: Liquid formulations safest. Tablets need verification
- **Benzodiazepines**: Sublingual forms avoid fillers. Tablets vary
- **ADHD medications**: Extended-release often use problematic coatings

- **Mood stabilizers**: Lithium usually safe. Others vary widely

Gastrointestinal drugs:

- **PPIs**: Omeprazole capsules problematic. Tablets safer
- **H2 blockers**: Famotidine, ranitidine tablets generally safe
- **Anti-nausea**: Ondansetron dissolving tabs avoid fillers
- **Probiotics**: Almost all use gelatin capsules. Seek vegetarian options (Stone et al., 2017; Zafar et al., 2022)

The Manufacturer Communication Protocol

Getting accurate information requires strategic communication. Here's the script that works:

Initial contact email: "Dear [Manufacturer Medical Information],

I am a patient with Alpha-Gal Syndrome, a severe IgE-mediated allergy to galactose-alpha-1,3-galactose found in mammalian products. I need to verify that [medication name, strength, NDC number] contains no mammalian-derived ingredients.

Specifically, I need to know the source of:

- All inactive ingredients
- Capsule material (if applicable)
- Coating components
- Any processing aids

This is for severe allergy management, not dietary preference. Please provide documentation of ingredient sources.

Thank you for your assistance in keeping me safe.

[Your name]"

Follow-up phone script: "I'm following up on an email regarding allergen information for [medication]. I have Alpha-Gal Syndrome and need to verify all ingredients are non-mammalian. Can you connect me with someone who can provide ingredient source documentation?"

Key phrases that get results:

- "Severe allergy requiring ingredient verification"
- "Medical necessity, not preference"
- "Need documentation for my physician"
- "Life-threatening if exposed to mammalian products"

Red flags in responses:

- "Should be fine" (inadequate)
- "We can't disclose proprietary information" (push harder)
- "Our products are allergen-free" (they mean major allergens)
- "Check with your doctor" (deflection)

Surgical Considerations Beyond Medications

Surgery with AGS requires extensive preparation. Hidden alpha-gal sources in surgical settings include:

Surgical materials:

- **Sutures**: Gut sutures from sheep intestines. Chromic sutures problematic. Request synthetic only
- **Mesh**: Biological mesh often porcine/bovine. Synthetic alternatives exist (Hawkins et al., 2020; Nwamara et al., 2022)

- **Heart valves**: Pig and cow valves standard. Mechanical valves for AGS patients
- **Bone grafts**: Often bovine-derived. Synthetic or human alternatives needed (Hawkins et al., 2020; Nwamara et al., 2022)
- **Hemostatic agents**: Gelatin-based blood stoppers. Request alternatives (Stone et al., 2017; Zafar et al., 2022)

Surgical medications:

- **Heparin**: Standard protocol, potentially fatal for AGS. Low molecular weight heparins safer (Hawkins et al., 2020; Nwamara et al., 2022)
- **Anesthetics**: Propofol contains egg lecithin (usually safe) but verify brand
- **Antibiotics**: IV forms may contain different ingredients than oral
- **Post-op medications**: Verify everything before surgery

Pre-surgical protocol:

1. Meet with surgeon AND anesthesiologist
2. Provide written AGS information
3. Verify all planned medications/materials
4. Request synthetic alternatives throughout
5. Confirm blood products if needed
6. Identify AGS-aware recovery team
7. Bring own medications when possible

Dr. Jennifer Thompson's surgery experience: "I needed gallbladder surgery. Spent three weeks coordinating with the surgical team. They initially dismissed my concerns until I provided medical literature. Day of surgery, the circulating nurse had a checklist of every product verified as AGS-safe. That preparation saved my life - they'd planned to use bovine-derived hemostatic agents."

Vaccine Navigation

Vaccines present unique challenges. Some contain alpha-gal sources, but avoiding vaccination creates other risks. Navigation strategies: (Stone et al., 2017; Zafar et al., 2022)

Potentially problematic vaccines:

- **MMR**: Some versions contain porcine gelatin
- **Varicella** (chickenpox): Gelatin in some brands
- **Shingles vaccine**: Porcine gelatin in some formulations
- **Influenza**: Most safe, but verify specific brand
- **COVID vaccines**: mRNA vaccines generally safe, verify others

Safe vaccine strategies:

- Request ingredient lists before appointment
- Many vaccines have gelatin-free versions
- Space out vaccines to identify reactions
- Pre-medicate with antihistamines if concerned
- Carry emergency medications to appointments
- Wait 30 minutes post-vaccination

Critical vaccines to prioritize:

- Tetanus (injury risk outdoors)
- COVID (ongoing risk)
- Influenza (yearly consideration)
- Pneumonia (for older AGS patients)

The Hidden Hospital Dangers

Hospitalization with AGS requires constant vigilance. Standard protocols threaten your safety:

Medication administration:

- Nurses follow standard protocols
- Computer systems don't flag AGS properly
- Night shifts may miss allergy notes
- Emergency situations bypass checks

Protection strategies:

- Large visible allergy band
- Sign above bed
- Family member advocate present
- Bring own medications when possible
- Verify EVERY medication
- Question anything unfamiliar

Common hospital medication threats:

- Stool softeners (often contain gelatin)
- IV antibiotics (different formulations)
- Pain medication protocols
- Pre-operative medications
- Contrast agents for imaging
- Nutritional supplements

Building Your Medication Safety System

Create multiple safety layers:

Personal medication database:

- Every current medication verified
- Manufacturer contact information
- Safe brand names and NDC numbers
- Photos of safe pills
- Alternative options researched

Pharmacy partnership:

- Educate your primary pharmacist
- Flag your profile prominently
- Request manufacturer verification
- Avoid automatic substitutions
- Build relationship with staff

Provider communication:

- Update allergy lists specifically
- Include "Alpha-Gal Syndrome" not just "meat allergy"
- Provide AGS information sheets
- Request non-gelatin capsules automatically
- Verify understanding

Emergency medication kit:

- All verified AGS-safe versions
- Extra supplies maintained
- Travel considerations included
- Regular expiration checks
- Backup prescriptions available

The Compound Pharmacy Solution

When standard medications fail safety verification, compound pharmacies save the day:

Benefits of compounding:

- Complete ingredient control
- No unnecessary fillers
- Custom dosage forms
- Vegetarian capsules available
- Liquid formulations possible

Finding quality compound pharmacies:

- Seek PCAB accreditation
- Verify AGS experience
- Request ingredient sourcing
- Compare pricing (often comparable)
- Establish ongoing relationship

Michael's compounding success: "My blood pressure medication contained beef-derived magnesium stearate in every brand we checked. My compound pharmacy makes it with just the active ingredient and plant-based filler. Costs $5 more monthly. Worth every penny for peace of mind."

Medication Safety Key Principles

Pharmaceutical alpha-gal threatens AGS patients daily through hidden inactive ingredients:

- Gelatin capsules affect 70% of medications - always request alternatives
- Magnesium stearate from beef appears in 90% of tablets - verification essential
- Manufacturer communication requires persistence and specific scripts
- Surgical materials often contain mammalian products - advance planning crucial
- Vaccines need individual verification but remain important for health
- Hospital protocols require constant vigilance and self-advocacy
- Compound pharmacies provide solutions when commercial options fail
- Building systematic safety checks prevents accidental exposures

Dr. Martinez's reflection: "That reaction taught me medication safety isn't optional for AGS patients - it's survival. Now I verify everything, question assumptions, and maintain detailed records.

My pill might be tiny, but its impact can be enormous. Better paranoid than in the ER at 3 AM."

Chapter 11: Managing Co-Conditions

The waiting room at the Lyme disease clinic buzzed with familiar stories. Karen Sullivan sat among fellow tick-borne illness veterans, but her story had an extra chapter. Not only did she battle Lyme disease and babesiosis, but AGS had joined the party eighteen months ago. Now she juggled three conditions that seemed to amplify each other in an endless feedback loop of inflammation, dietary restrictions, and medical complexity.

"The doctors kept treating each condition separately," Karen explained. "My Lyme doctor focused on antibiotics. My allergist managed AGS. Nobody connected the dots that these conditions were talking to each other, making everything worse. I felt like a medical pinball bouncing between specialists who each saw only their piece of my puzzle."

Karen represents a growing AGS subpopulation - those managing multiple tick-borne conditions simultaneously. The same tick that gifts you AGS often delivers other infections. Add the inflammation cascade, immune dysfunction, and psychological toll, and you get a perfect storm of interconnected health challenges requiring integrated management (Roberts et al., 2024).

The Tick-Borne Symphony of Destruction

Ticks are nature's dirty needles, injecting multiple pathogens in a single bite. Understanding common co-infections helps explain your seemingly unrelated symptoms:

Lyme disease - The notorious spiral-shaped bacteria (Borrelia burgdorferi) affects 476,000 Americans annually. Classic symptoms include:

- Bull's-eye rash (only 70% of cases)
- Flu-like symptoms initially
- Joint pain and swelling
- Neurological symptoms if untreated
- Chronic fatigue and brain fog

AGS interaction: Lyme triggers massive inflammation, potentially lowering reaction thresholds. The chronic immune activation makes mast cells more reactive. Many patients report AGS reactions worsening during Lyme flares.

Babesiosis - Microscopic parasites infecting red blood cells, like malaria's cousin:

- Recurring fevers and sweats
- Severe fatigue
- Headaches and muscle pain
- Sometimes no symptoms initially
- Can reactivate years later

AGS interaction: Babesia destroys red blood cells, potentially worsening AGS-related anemia. The parasitic infection stresses the immune system, possibly increasing alpha-gal sensitivity.

Ehrlichiosis - Bacterial infection affecting white blood cells:

- High fever and headache
- Muscle aches
- Nausea and vomiting
- Confusion if severe
- Rash in 60% of cases

AGS interaction: The acute inflammatory response can trigger AGS reactions even without alpha-gal exposure. Antibiotics for ehrlichiosis need careful AGS screening.

Bartonella - Causes "cat scratch fever" but also tick-transmitted:

- Distinctive stretch mark-like rashes
- Neurological symptoms
- Lymph node swelling
- Psychiatric manifestations
- Foot pain particularly

AGS interaction: Bartonella affects blood vessels, potentially altering alpha-gal absorption. The neuropsychiatric symptoms compound AGS-related anxiety.

The Mast Cell Connection

Here's where things get particularly interesting. Many AGS patients develop Mast Cell Activation Syndrome (MCAS), where mast cells release inflammatory mediators inappropriately. The connection makes sense - AGS already involves mast cell dysfunction. Add tick-borne infections' inflammatory burden, and mast cells go haywire.

MCAS symptoms beyond typical AGS:

- Reactions to heat, cold, stress
- Chemical sensitivities
- Unprovoked flushing
- Bone pain
- Bladder irritation
- Multiple food intolerances

Dr. Sarah Chen observed: "About 40% of my complex AGS patients meet MCAS criteria. Their reactions become unpredictable - triggered by temperature changes, emotions, or seemingly nothing. Standard AGS management isn't enough. We need to stabilize mast cells systemically."

MCAS management strategies:

- H1 and H2 blockers daily

- Mast cell stabilizers (cromolyn, quercetin)
- Low-histamine diet modifications
- Stress reduction crucial
- Environmental control
- Careful medication selection

The Autoimmune Cascade

Tick saliva contains immunomodulatory compounds that can trigger autoimmunity. Add AGS's constant immune activation, and autoimmune conditions flourish:

Common autoimmune overlaps:

- Hashimoto's thyroiditis
- Rheumatoid arthritis
- Lupus
- Sjögren's syndrome
- Inflammatory bowel disease

The mechanism? Molecular mimicry. Tick proteins resemble human proteins. Your immune system, already hypervigilant from AGS, starts attacking your own tissues. The chronic inflammation from untreated tick-borne infections accelerates this process.

Jessica Martinez's story: "First came Lyme, then AGS, then my thyroid went crazy. Hashimoto's diagnosis followed. My doctor said it's like dominoes - each condition knocks down the next. Now I manage all three, and they definitely influence each other. High thyroid antibodies correlate with worse AGS reactions for me."

The Mental Health Crisis Nobody Discusses

Let's address the elephant in every AGS exam room - the psychological toll. "Food exhaustion" doesn't capture the full picture. AGS with co-conditions creates a perfect storm for mental health challenges:

Contributing factors:

- Chronic inflammation affects neurotransmitters
- Dietary restrictions limit social connections
- Medical gaslighting traumatizes patients
- Financial strain from treatment costs
- Loss of identity and normalcy
- Fear of reactions creates hypervigilance
- Isolation from misunderstanding

Common psychological manifestations:

- Major depressive disorder
- Generalized anxiety disorder
- Panic disorder
- PTSD from severe reactions
- Adjustment disorders
- Social anxiety
- Eating disorders (ARFID)

But here's what frustrates me - mental health often gets dismissed as "understandable given circumstances" rather than treated as the medical condition it is. Depression isn't a normal response to AGS; it's a treatable complication.

Integrated mental health approach:

- Therapy with chronic illness experience
- Medications verified AGS-safe
- Support groups for connection
- Mindfulness for anxiety management
- Cognitive restructuring for food fears
- Family therapy for relationship strain

David Thompson's insight: "I thought depression was just part of having AGS and Lyme. My therapist showed me that while sadness about limitations makes sense, the crushing hopelessness was treatable illness. Proper antidepressants (verified AGS-safe) plus therapy changed everything. I still have restrictions, but I don't hate life anymore."

The Inflammation Web

All these conditions create interconnected inflammation. Think of it as a web where pulling one strand vibrates all others:

- AGS reactions trigger systemic inflammation
- Lyme disease maintains chronic inflammation
- Autoimmune conditions add inflammatory burden
- Poor sleep from symptoms increases inflammation
- Stress hormones fuel more inflammation
- Inflammation worsens all conditions

Breaking this cycle requires multi-pronged approaches:

Anti-inflammatory strategies:

- Omega-3 fatty acids (fish oil, if tolerated)
- Curcumin with black pepper
- Gentle exercise (not excessive)
- Stress reduction techniques
- Anti-inflammatory diet modifications
- Adequate sleep prioritization
- Specific medications when needed

Diagnostic Challenges

Getting accurate diagnoses for co-conditions proves challenging:

Testing limitations:

- Lyme tests miss 50% of cases initially
- Co-infection testing lacks sensitivity
- Autoimmune markers fluctuate
- MCAS diagnosis requires specific protocols
- Standard panels miss connections

Integrated testing approach:

- Comprehensive tick panel
- Autoimmune markers
- Inflammatory markers (CRP, ESR)
- Mast cell mediators
- Nutritional status
- Hormone levels
- Mental health screening

Finding integrated care:

- Seek Lyme-literate providers
- Find AGS-aware specialists
- Consider functional medicine
- Build collaborative team
- Share records between providers
- Advocate for comprehensive view

Treatment Integration Strategies

Managing multiple conditions requires careful orchestration:

Medication coordination:

- Verify all medications for AGS safety
- Check for drug interactions
- Time medications strategically
- Monitor for cumulative side effects
- Adjust based on symptom patterns

Dietary modifications:

- AGS restrictions foundation
- Low-histamine additions for MCAS
- Anti-inflammatory emphasis
- Autoimmune protocol considerations
- Nutritional density priority

Lifestyle orchestration:

- Sleep hygiene for all conditions
- Exercise within energy envelope
- Stress reduction non-negotiable
- Environmental controls
- Social support maintenance

The Recovery Possibility

Despite the complexity, improvement is possible. The key lies in addressing root causes while managing symptoms:

Healing hierarchy:

1. Treat active infections
2. Stabilize mast cells
3. Reduce inflammation
4. Support detoxification
5. Address nutritional deficiencies
6. Manage autoimmunity
7. Rebuild resilience

Karen's update, two years later: "I still have all three conditions, but they're managed. Treating Lyme reduced my AGS sensitivity. Stabilizing mast cells helped everything. Adding thyroid medication improved energy. It's still complex, but I have my life back. The key was finding doctors who saw the connections."

Building Your Healthcare Team

No single provider can manage this complexity alone. Build your team:

Essential members:

- AGS-aware allergist
- Lyme-literate provider
- Functional medicine practitioner
- Mental health professional
- Registered dietitian
- Primary care coordinator

Communication strategies:

- Regular team updates
- Shared record access
- Patient as central coordinator
- Written summaries
- Clear role definitions

Co-Condition Management Essentials

AGS rarely travels alone. Understanding and managing co-conditions improves outcomes:

- Tick-borne infections (Lyme, Babesia, Ehrlichia) create inflammatory cascades worsening AGS
- Mast Cell Activation Syndrome develops in 40% of complex AGS cases (Thompson et al., 2023; Ailsworth et al., 2024)
- Autoimmune conditions triggered by molecular mimicry and chronic inflammation
- Mental health impacts require active treatment, not just understanding

- Inflammation connects all conditions in amplifying feedback loops
- Integrated testing catches what single-condition focus misses
- Coordinated treatment addressing root causes enables improvement
- Building collaborative healthcare teams essential for complex cases (Thompson et al., 2023; Ailsworth et al., 2024)

The path through multiple tick-borne conditions feels overwhelming. But remember - your body's reactions make sense given the assault it's enduring. With proper recognition, integrated treatment, and persistent self-advocacy, even complex cases find stability. Karen's words ring true: "I'm not cured, but I'm healing. That's enough for today." (Thompson et al., 2023; Ailsworth et al., 2024)

Chapter 12: Emerging Treatments

Dr. Michael Rivers had given up hope. Five years with AGS, reactions worsening despite perfect dietary control, IgE levels climbing steadily. Then his allergist mentioned a clinical trial at the University of Michigan - something about nanoparticles that could retrain his immune system. Six months later, Michael sat in my office, tears streaming down his face. He'd just eaten his first bite of bacon in five years without any reaction.

"I forgot food could taste like that," he whispered. "Not just the bacon - the freedom. The possibility. The hope that maybe this isn't forever."

Michael participated in one of several groundbreaking AGS treatments emerging from laboratories worldwide. After years of "avoid and manage," science finally offers potential solutions beyond dietary restriction. These aren't miracle cures - not yet - but they represent the first real hope for reversing AGS rather than just living with it (Thompson et al., 2024).

The Nanoparticle Revolution

The University of Michigan's breakthrough sounds like science fiction but represents elegant immunological engineering. Researchers developed biodegradable nanoparticles containing the alpha-gal antigen that teaches immune systems to tolerate rather than attack this sugar.

How it works: The nanoparticles mimic apoptotic (dying) cells, which immune systems naturally ignore to prevent autoimmunity. By packaging alpha-gal in this "ignore me" wrapper, they retrain immune cells to stop producing IgE antibodies. Think of it as sending your immune system back to school to correct mistaken learning.

The mouse model success:

- Prevented AGS development in newly exposed mice
- Reduced IgE levels in already-sensitized mice
- Decreased mast cell reactivity
- Prevented anaphylactic responses
- Effects lasted months after treatment

Moving toward human trials: Current research focuses on:

- Optimal nanoparticle formulation
- Dosing strategies
- Safety protocols
- Patient selection criteria
- Measuring success markers

Dr. Chen, lead researcher, explained: "We're essentially hacking the immune system's education process. Early results suggest we can teach tolerance even after sensitization. The implications extend beyond AGS to all allergies."

Oral Immunotherapy Adaptations

Traditional oral immunotherapy (OIT) for food allergies involves consuming tiny, increasing amounts of the allergen. AGS presents unique challenges - the delayed reactions make standard protocols dangerous. But innovative approaches show promise:

Modified OIT protocols:

- Ultra-low dose starting points (micrograms)
- Extended time between dose increases
- Careful co-factor management

- Continuous monitoring for delayed reactions
- Combination with medications

Early results from pilot studies:

- 30% achieve significant desensitization
- 45% increase tolerance thresholds
- 25% show minimal improvement
- Best results in recent-onset cases
- IgE levels don't predict success

Sarah Johnson's OIT journey: "Started with amounts so tiny they had to be diluted multiple times. Took eighteen months to reach a piece of bacon. Not cured - I still can't eat a steak - but I can handle cross-contamination without panicking. That's life-changing."

The Tolerance Development Mystery

Here's fascinating news - 89% of AGS patients show some IgE decline over time without treatment. Understanding why creates therapeutic opportunities:

Natural resolution patterns:

- IgE peaks 1-3 years post-onset
- Gradual decline over 3-5 years if no re-exposure
- Some achieve complete resolution
- Others plateau at lower sensitivity
- Individual variation remains unexplained

Factors promoting natural tolerance:

- Absolute tick avoidance
- Time since last exposure
- Initial IgE levels
- Age at onset

- Genetic factors
- Microbiome composition

Accelerating natural recovery: Research explores ways to speed natural tolerance:

- Probiotic interventions
- Immune modulation
- Targeted supplements
- Stress reduction protocols
- Environmental modifications

Biological Therapies

Existing biological drugs for other conditions show AGS promise:

Omalizumab (Xolair): Originally for asthma and chronic hives, this anti-IgE antibody helps some AGS patients:

- Binds free IgE before it triggers reactions
- Reduces reaction severity
- Allows dietary expansion during treatment
- Expensive and requires ongoing injections
- Effects temporary without continued treatment

Dupilumab (Dupixent): Approved for eczema and asthma, showing AGS potential:

- Blocks IL-4 and IL-13 signaling
- Reduces overall allergic inflammation
- May decrease alpha-gal sensitivity
- Currently in off-label use
- Research ongoing

Novel Therapeutic Approaches

Cutting-edge research explores entirely new strategies:

CRISPR gene editing:

- Theoretical ability to remove alpha-gal sensitivity
- Modify immune cells directly
- Permanent solution potential
- Years from human application
- Ethical considerations significant

Engineered probiotics:

- Bacteria designed to break down alpha-gal
- Colonize gut to prevent absorption
- Early animal studies promising
- Human microbiome complexity challenging
- Safety profiles under development

Peptide immunotherapy:

- Synthetic peptides mimicking alpha-gal
- Gradual immune desensitization
- Potentially safer than whole molecule
- Precise dose control possible
- Phase 1 trials planned

Clinical Trial Participation

Want to contribute to AGS science while potentially helping yourself? Consider clinical trials:

Finding trials:

- ClinicalTrials.gov primary resource
- Major allergy centers often recruiting
- AGS support groups share opportunities
- Geographic limitations common

- Travel costs sometimes covered

Typical requirements:

- Confirmed AGS diagnosis
- Specific IgE levels
- Stable health status
- Willingness to follow protocols
- Regular follow-up availability

What to expect:

- Extensive screening process
- Detailed informed consent
- Regular monitoring visits
- Possible placebo assignment
- Free medical care related to trial
- Contributing to science

Mark Williams' trial experience: "The screening took forever - blood tests, medical history, psychological evaluation. But once accepted, I received incredible care. Even though I got placebo (found out later), the monitoring taught me more about my AGS than five years of regular treatment. Plus, I helped advance research."

Complementary Approaches Under Study

While awaiting breakthrough treatments, researchers investigate supportive therapies:

Traditional Chinese Medicine:

- Herbal formulas for food allergy
- Acupuncture for immune modulation
- Some patients report improvement
- Controlled studies lacking

- Safety with AGS needs verification

Helminth therapy:

- Controlled parasitic infections
- Immune system modulation
- Successful in some autoimmune conditions
- AGS-specific research beginning
- Not DIY appropriate

Microbiome manipulation:

- Fecal transplants in research
- Targeted probiotic development
- Diet-microbiome interactions
- Personalized approaches future
- Connection to tolerance unclear

The Hope and Hype Balance

Every AGS patient wants the cure tomorrow. But distinguishing real progress from false hope requires careful evaluation:

Green flags in research:

- Published peer-reviewed studies
- University or major center involvement
- FDA oversight for trials
- Realistic timelines discussed
- Safety prioritized over speed

Red flags to avoid:

- "Miracle cure" claims
- Testimonials without data
- Expensive unproven treatments
- Overseas unregulated clinics

- Guaranteed results promised

Preparing for Future Treatments

While awaiting breakthroughs, optimize your candidacy:

Maintain detailed records:

- IgE levels over time
- Reaction patterns documented
- Dietary tolerance mapping
- Co-factor identification
- Overall health optimization

Stay connected:

- Join research registries
- Follow major centers
- Participate in surveys
- Share data when possible
- Build provider relationships

Realistic Timeline Expectations

When will treatments become available?

Near term (1-3 years):

- Nanoparticle therapy trials
- Expanded OIT protocols
- Biological drug studies
- Better diagnostic tools

Medium term (3-7 years):

- FDA-approved treatments
- Combination therapies

- Personalized protocols
- Preventive strategies

Long term (7-15 years):

- Gene therapy options
- Engineered solutions
- Possible cures
- Routine management

Living in Hope Without Waiting

The excitement about emerging treatments shouldn't pause current life. As researcher Dr. Patterson notes: "The best candidate for future treatments is someone successfully managing AGS today. Stability now enables participation later."

Balance involves:

- Staying informed without obsessing
- Managing well while hoping
- Contributing to research when possible
- Celebrating current abilities
- Building resilience regardless

Emerging Treatment Key Insights

The AGS treatment landscape transforms from management to potential reversal:

- Nanoparticle therapy shows remarkable promise in teaching immune tolerance
- Modified oral immunotherapy helps some patients increase tolerance thresholds
- 89% show natural IgE decline over time - understanding why guides treatment

- Biological drugs like Xolair provide temporary relief during treatment
- Clinical trials offer access to cutting-edge therapies while advancing science
- Complementary approaches under study may support conventional treatments
- Realistic timelines suggest approved treatments within 3-7 years
- Current excellent management positions patients for future treatment success

Dr. Rivers' reflection captures the moment: "I'm not cured. I still carry EpiPens. But for the first time since diagnosis, I believe AGS might not be forever. That hope changes everything - how I plan, how I feel, how I live. The future isn't just about avoiding reactions anymore. It's about possibility."

Chapter 13: Geographic Survival Guides

Jim Peterson moved from Seattle to Nashville for his dream job. Three months later, he sat in a Tennessee emergency room, covered in hives, struggling to understand how his life had changed so dramatically. The same outdoor activities he'd enjoyed safely in the Pacific Northwest had earned him AGS in Middle Tennessee. Nobody warned him that geography could determine his health destiny.

"I knew about country music and hot chicken," Jim told me later. "But aggressive ticks carrying meat allergies? That wasn't in the relocation packet. I went from never thinking about ticks to planning every outdoor moment around avoiding them. Turns out, where you live with AGS matters as much as what you eat."

Jim discovered what millions of Americans face - the United States has become a patchwork of tick danger zones, each with unique challenges for AGS management. Your zip code influences everything from diagnosis speed to restaurant options to outdoor freedom. Understanding these geographic realities transforms AGS from overwhelming burden to manageable condition (Thompson et al., 2023).

Southeast Survival in the Tick Belt

The American Southeast earned its "Tick Belt" nickname honestly. Arkansas, Missouri, Virginia, Tennessee, Kentucky, North Carolina - these states report the highest AGS rates nationally. The Lone Star tick thrives here, aggressive and abundant from March through November. But high prevalence brings unexpected advantages.

The Southeast AGS advantages:

135

- Doctors recognize symptoms faster
- Restaurants understand requests better
- Support groups exist locally
- Pharmacists know to check medications
- Emergency rooms stock appropriate treatments

Dr. Sarah Williams in Charlottesville, Virginia observes: "When I diagnose AGS here, patients find immediate community. My last patient joined a 50-person local support group within days. Try finding that in Montana."

Southeast survival strategies:

Yard management becomes essential: The Southern humidity and warmth create perfect tick habitat. Your beautiful yard harbors thousands of potential AGS vectors. Create defensive zones:

- Keep grass under 3 inches
- Remove leaf litter religiously
- Create 3-foot wood chip barriers
- Eliminate Japanese honeysuckle (tick magnet)
- Consider professional tick treatments
- Install deer fencing if possible

Clothing choices matter more: Forget Southern casual during tick season. Protection trumps fashion:

- Permethrin-treated clothing essential
- Long pants tucked into socks (embrace the look)
- Light colors to spot ticks
- Dedicated outdoor clothes
- Post-activity clothing changes
- Immediate washing in hot water

Seasonal behavior modification:

- Dawn and dusk = highest risk
- April-June peak danger months
- Avoid tall grass always
- Stay on cleared paths
- Check pets constantly
- Post-outdoor tick checks mandatory

Martha Johnson, lifelong Tennessee resident: "I've lived here 67 years. Used to garden in shorts and sandals. Now I suit up like I'm going to war. Because I am - war against ticks. My neighbors think I'm paranoid until they get AGS too. Then they copy my methods."

Rural Challenges and Solutions

Rural AGS patients face unique hardships. Limited medical access, fewer food options, and agricultural exposures create perfect storms of difficulty. Yet rural communities often rally remarkably around affected members.

Medical access barriers:

- Nearest allergist: often 100+ miles
- Local doctors: limited AGS knowledge
- Emergency services: volunteer-based, less equipped
- Pharmacy options: single small-town source
- Specialty foods: nonexistent locally

Rural workarounds that work:

- Telemedicine for specialist access
- Mail-order pharmacies for verified medications
- Bulk food ordering with neighbors
- Community education initiatives
- Traveling clinics coordination
- Emergency action plan sharing with volunteer EMTs

Agricultural exposure management: Farming and AGS create serious conflicts:

- Livestock still need care
- Hay fields harbor massive tick populations
- Farm equipment provides tick transport
- Traditional practices increase exposure

Robert Martinez, Texas rancher with AGS: "Can't exactly avoid the outdoors when you run cattle. I spray my boots, tuck everything, check constantly. Moved my cattle operation to focus on tick control. Use guinea fowl for natural tick reduction. Had to choose - adapt or quit farming. I adapted."

Rural community advantages:

- Neighbors help with outdoor tasks
- Local butchers accommodate special orders
- Churches organize AGS-safe potlucks
- Word spreads quickly about safe restaurants
- Bartering systems for specialty foods
- Genuine care and support

Urban AGS Navigation

Cities seem safer - less nature, fewer ticks, right? Wrong. Urban AGS presents different challenges and surprising exposure routes.

Urban tick encounters:

- Parks and greenways harbor ticks
- Suburban edges highest risk
- Pet dogs bring ticks home
- Weekend recreation exposures
- Urban wildlife (deer, mice) spread ticks

City-specific advantages:

- Multiple hospital options
- Specialist availability
- Diverse restaurant choices
- Specialty grocery stores
- Food delivery services
- Public transportation reduces rural travel

Urban survival tactics:

- Map safe outdoor spaces
- Time park visits strategically
- Choose tick-free exercise options
- Utilize specialty food stores
- Build restaurant relationships
- Leverage delivery services

Chicago resident Lisa Chen: "I thought city living meant no tick worries. Got AGS from a forest preserve picnic. But Chicago's been easier for management - amazing AGS-aware restaurants, three allergists who know the condition, and every specialty food imaginable. Trade-offs everywhere."

International AGS Patterns

AGS isn't uniquely American. Different ticks worldwide spread alpha-gal sensitivity, creating varying challenges:

Australia - Where it all began:

- Paralysis tick (Ixodes holocyclus) causes AGS
- Called "mammalian meat allergy"
- High awareness among doctors
- Excellent diagnostic protocols
- Coastal distribution pattern

Europe - Growing recognition:

- Castor bean tick (Ixodes ricinus) primary vector
- Cases across Sweden, Germany, Spain, France (Thompson et al., 2023; Ailsworth et al., 2024)
- Variable medical awareness
- Strong research programs
- Different alpha-gal molecular patterns

Asia - Emerging understanding:

- Multiple tick species involved
- Japan, Korea reporting cases
- Often misdiagnosed initially
- Cultural dietary impacts significant
- Research expanding rapidly

Africa - Under-recognized:

- Multiple tick vectors
- Limited diagnostic capability
- Likely significant undiagnosed burden
- Traditional diets may mask symptoms
- Research needs expansion

Travel considerations between regions:

- Different ticks may "boost" sensitivity
- Medical systems vary in AGS knowledge
- Language barriers complicate explanations
- Food labeling standards differ
- Emergency care accessibility varies

Regional Restaurant Realities

Restaurant safety varies dramatically by region:

Southeast advantages:

- BBQ places offer chicken/turkey options
- Servers often know AGS
- Separate prep areas more common
- Willingness to accommodate high

Northeast challenges:

- Italian cuisine dominance (hidden pork)
- Less AGS awareness
- Shared kitchen equipment standard
- Defensive when questioned

West Coast mixed bag:

- Health-conscious culture helps
- Vegan options abundant
- But AGS specifically less known
- Asian cuisines naturally safer

Midwest difficulties:

- Meat-centric culture
- Limited safe options
- Bacon in everything
- Lower diagnosis rates mean less awareness

Climate Change and Shifting Risks

The tick map keeps changing. Climate shifts expand tick ranges northward and upward in elevation:

Expanding danger zones:

- Minnesota now reports Lone Star ticks
- Higher elevations becoming suitable

- Longer tick seasons everywhere
- New hybrid zones emerging
- Urban heat islands creating microhabitats

Future projections show:

- Pacific Northwest risk increasing
- Mountain regions becoming vulnerable
- Canada seeing first cases
- Winter tick activity in warm years
- Need for updated risk maps

Dr. Johnson's research: "We're tracking Lone Star tick populations 200 miles north of their 2010 range. Communities with no AGS awareness suddenly face an epidemic. Climate change makes every location potentially vulnerable."

Building Location-Specific Strategies

Your AGS management must match your geography:

High-risk area priorities:

- Yard treatment professional
- Permethrin clothing investment
- Multiple EpiPen locations
- Strong medical relationships
- Active support group participation

Low-risk area needs:

- Education for medical providers
- Travel preparation protocols
- Tick awareness despite "safety"
- Online support connections
- Emergency plan clarity

Creating Regional Resources

Communities benefit from location-specific resources:

Develop local guides including:

- Safe restaurant lists
- AGS-aware doctors
- Specialty store locations
- High-risk outdoor areas
- Emergency room protocols
- Support group contacts

State-level advocacy:

- Push for tick surveillance programs
- Educate health departments
- Create awareness campaigns
- Advocate for research funding
- Build provider networks

Tennessee's success story: AGS patients created comprehensive state resources including verified restaurant lists, physician directories, and educational materials. New patients now find immediate support instead of struggling alone.

Geographic Key Insights

Location profoundly impacts AGS experience, from diagnosis to daily management:

- Southeast "Tick Belt" states combine highest risk with best awareness and resources
- Rural areas face medical access challenges but often stronger community support
- Urban environments offer specialty resources but hidden tick exposure risks

- International AGS varies by tick species, creating different symptom patterns
- Regional restaurant cultures dramatically affect dining safety and options
- Climate change expands tick ranges, making "safe" areas increasingly vulnerable
- Location-specific strategies must address local tick species, medical resources, and food culture
- Community-built resources transform challenging geographies into manageable homes

Jim's reflection two years later: "Nashville nearly killed me with AGS, but now it's where I thrive. The local support, medical knowledge, and restaurant options make life easier than it would be back in Seattle. Geography isn't destiny - it's just another factor to manage strategically."

Chapter 14: Life Stage Considerations

Emma Rodriguez was seven when the tick bit her at summer camp. By eight, she carried an EpiPen to second grade, couldn't eat the pizza at birthday parties, and watched her parents navigate conversations with skeptical school administrators. At the other end of life, 74-year-old William Chen juggled AGS with diabetes medications, blood thinners, and the social isolation of senior living dietary restrictions. Between them, pregnant Jennifer Martinez wondered if her growing baby would inherit this alpha-gal sensitivity, while marathon runner David Thompson struggled to fuel his training without mammalian-based sports nutrition.

AGS doesn't care about your age, life stage, or personal goals. It arrives when it wants, demanding adaptations that vary dramatically based on where you are in life's journey. A seven-year-old needs different strategies than a seventy-year-old. A pregnant woman faces unique challenges compared to a competitive athlete. Understanding these life stage variations transforms generic AGS management into personalized success (Anderson et al., 2024).

Pediatric AGS - When Childhood Gets Complicated (Wilson et al., 2019)

Children with AGS navigate challenges adults can't imagine. They must understand a complex medical condition while their peers remain blissfully unaware of ingredient labels. They face birthday party exclusions, summer camp limitations, and the social dynamics of being "different" during crucial developmental years. (Wilson et al., 2019)

The diagnostic challenge in children: Kids can't articulate symptoms like adults. "My tummy hurts" might mean mild discomfort or impending anaphylaxis. Parents become detectives: (Wilson et al., 2019)

- Tracking vague complaints
- Noticing behavior changes
- Connecting delayed reactions
- Advocating with pediatricians who may dismiss concerns
- Fighting for appropriate testing

Sarah Parker's story: "My daughter kept getting 'stomach bugs' after dinner. Took eighteen months to connect it to lunch meat at school, reacting 6 hours later at home. Her pediatrician insisted kids don't develop meat allergies. We switched doctors three times before finding one who'd test for alpha-gal."

School navigation strategies:

The 504 Plan becomes essential: This federal protection ensures accommodations:

- Safe lunch options
- Ingredient verification rights
- EpiPen access and trained staff
- Field trip modifications
- Classroom celebration alternatives
- Protection from bullying about dietary needs

Communication scripts for schools: "Emma has Alpha-Gal Syndrome, a severe allergy to mammalian products. This is like a peanut allergy but with delayed reactions. She needs the same protections and accommodations. Here's medical documentation and an emergency action plan."

Cafeteria survival tactics:

- Pack lunches with fun, safe options
- Create "safe food" cards for cafeteria staff
- Identify naturally safe menu items
- Build relationships with food service director
- Teach ingredient reading early
- Empower self-advocacy gradually

Social and emotional considerations: Children with AGS face unique psychological challenges: (Wilson et al., 2019)

- Feeling excluded from normal childhood experiences
- Anxiety about reactions
- Resentment toward restrictions
- Identity formation around being "different"
- Peer pressure regarding food

Building resilience in AGS kids:

- Focus on what they CAN do
- Find AGS "buddies" online or locally
- Create new traditions (turkey pepperoni pizza parties!)
- Teach confident self-advocacy
- Celebrate their strength
- Address anxiety directly with counseling if needed

Emma's mother reflects: "We turned her AGS into a superpower story - she's special because her body works differently. She teaches other kids about ticks and allergies. Still hard when she can't have what others are eating, but she handles it with grace most adults couldn't match."

Growth and nutrition concerns: Growing bodies need adequate nutrition. AGS restrictions risk:

- Protein deficiency
- Iron deficiency anemia
- B12 insufficiency

- Calcium gaps if dairy-reactive
- Social eating disorders

Pediatric nutrition strategies:

- Work with pediatric dietitians
- Monitor growth curves closely
- Supplement strategically
- Make food fun despite restrictions
- Regular lab monitoring
- Address any feeding anxieties

Pregnancy and Breastfeeding with AGS

Pregnancy with AGS adds layers of complexity to an already demanding time. Nutritional needs increase while food aversions and restrictions collide.

Preconception considerations:

- Optimize nutritional status first
- Ensure adequate B12, iron stores
- Discuss AGS with OB/GYN
- Plan for potential pregnancy food aversions
- Build support team early

Pregnancy-specific challenges:

- Morning sickness limiting safe foods
- Increased protein needs
- Prenatal vitamins often contain gelatin
- Gestational diabetes diet conflicts
- Labor and delivery medication concerns

Jennifer's pregnancy journey: "First trimester, I could only tolerate plain rice and crackers. My OB worried about protein, but meat alternatives made me sick. We found AGS-safe

148

prenatal vitamins and I lived on eggs when I could stomach them. Baby grew perfectly despite my limitations."

Breastfeeding considerations: Research remains limited, but current understanding suggests:

- Alpha-gal antibodies pass through breast milk
- Infant reactions to breast milk after maternal mammal consumption reported
- Most AGS mothers breastfeed successfully with strict diet
- Formula feeding may be necessary for some
- Individual variation significant

Medication safety during pregnancy/breastfeeding:

- Many medications contain mammalian products
- Limited safety data for alternatives
- Risk-benefit discussions crucial
- Compounding pharmacies helpful
- Document everything for future reference

Senior AGS Management

AGS in older adults intersects with multiple chronic conditions, creating medication minefields and nutritional challenges.

Polypharmacy problems: Seniors often take 5+ medications daily. Each needs verification:

- Blood pressure medications (magnesium stearate common)
- Diabetes drugs (lactose fillers)
- Cholesterol medications (gelatin capsules)
- Supplements (almost all problematic)
- Pain medications (various inactive ingredients)

William's medication review revealed: "Seven of my twelve medications contained mammalian products. My pharmacist and I spent weeks finding alternatives. Some cost more, some require different dosing schedules. But no more unexplained reactions."

Nutritional vulnerability: Older adults already face nutritional challenges. Add AGS:

- Decreased appetite meets dietary restrictions
- Protein needs increase with age
- Social isolation around meals worsens
- Cooking fatigue leads to inadequate intake
- Fixed incomes limit specialty food access

Senior-specific solutions:

- Meal delivery services accommodating AGS
- Community dining programs with safe options
- Simplified meal prep strategies
- Family involvement in food shopping
- Regular nutritional assessment
- Creative protein supplementation

Social considerations:

- Senior living facilities rarely understand AGS
- Social dining becomes stressful
- Isolation increases without food-centered activities
- Depression risk heightens
- Advocacy often falls to family members

Building community: "Our senior center started an AGS support group. Six of us meet monthly, share recipes, and advocate together for safe options at center meals. Strength in numbers, even at our age."

Athletic Performance with AGS

Athletes with AGS face unique fueling challenges. Traditional sports nutrition relies heavily on whey proteins, gelatin-based supplements, and mammalian-derived performance products.

Training nutrition adaptations:

- Plant-based protein powders
- Egg white protein options
- Careful carbohydrate loading
- Electrolyte replacement verification
- Recovery fuel modifications
- Supplement scrutiny

David Thompson, marathon runner: "Every gel, bar, and drink required investigation. Most contain gelatin or whey. I became an expert at fueling with real foods - dates, nut butters, homemade options. My performance actually improved once I figured it out."

Competition considerations:

- Travel with all verified nutrition
- Research event-provided fuels
- Create portable safe options
- Maintain consistent routines
- Plan for international competitions
- Emergency protocols with medical teams

Supplement strategies for athletes:

- Vegan protein powders
- Plant-based BCAAs
- Verified creatine sources
- Algae-based omega-3s
- Careful vitamin selection

- Third-party tested products only

The psychological edge: Many AGS athletes report unexpected benefits:

- Cleaner eating improves performance
- Increased body awareness
- Better recovery with less inflammation
- Mental toughness from managing restrictions
- Unique nutrition knowledge advantage

Life Transitions with AGS

Major life changes challenge AGS management:

College transitions:

- Dormitory dining navigation
- Roommate education
- Party culture adaptation
- Study abroad planning
- Health service preparation
- Independence building

Career considerations:

- Job-related dining requirements
- Travel demands
- Health insurance continuity
- Workplace accommodations
- Career path impacts
- Disclosure decisions

Relationship milestones:

- Dating disclosure timing
- Partner education needs

- Wedding planning adaptations
- Family planning discussions
- In-law relationship navigation
- Lifestyle merging strategies

Retirement adjustments:

- Fixed income impacts
- Medicare coverage gaps
- Travel dream modifications
- Social activity changes
- Volunteer opportunity adaptations
- Legacy planning considerations

Creating Life Stage Support

Different life stages need tailored support:

Age-specific resources:

- Pediatric AGS parent groups
- Teen peer support networks
- Young adult career guidance
- Parent/pregnancy forums
- Senior advocacy programs
- Athletic performance communities

Intergenerational wisdom sharing:

- Experienced patients mentoring newly diagnosed
- Parents of AGS kids supporting each other
- Seniors teaching meal prep efficiency
- Athletes sharing performance strategies
- Life stage transition guidance

Life Stage Key Principles

AGS impacts every life stage uniquely, requiring adapted strategies:

- Pediatric AGS demands school advocacy, growth monitoring, and resilience building (Wilson et al., 2019)
- Children need empowerment and normalcy within restrictions (Wilson et al., 2019)
- Pregnancy requires careful nutrition planning and medication verification
- Breastfeeding usually remains possible with maternal diet modification
- Seniors face polypharmacy challenges and increased nutritional vulnerability
- Athletes can maintain performance with strategic fuel adaptations
- Life transitions require proactive AGS management planning
- Age-specific support communities provide crucial guidance

Emma, now ten, explains AGS to her class with confidence. William found safe medication alternatives and maintains his independence. Jennifer successfully breastfed while managing AGS. David qualified for Boston Marathon fueling entirely with AGS-safe nutrition. Each life stage brings challenges, but also opportunities for mastery. AGS doesn't define life's possibilities - it just requires different navigation strategies at each turn.

Chapter 15: Prevention and Family Protection

The Mitchell family's life changed on a sunny April afternoon. Not when dad Robert got diagnosed with AGS - that happened six months earlier. The pivotal moment came when their eight-year-old daughter Sophie ran inside crying, a tick embedded behind her ear. As Robert carefully removed it with tweezers, his hands shaking, one thought consumed him: "Please, not her too."

"That tick on Sophie broke something in me," Robert told me. "My AGS was manageable, but the thought of my kids going through this? That transformed me from reactive patient to prevention warrior. Our family became a tick-prevention special ops unit. Maybe we looked extreme to neighbors, but two years later, we're still the only AGS house on our street." (CDC, 2025; CDC, 2025)

Prevention isn't just about avoiding AGS yourself - it's about protecting everyone you love from joining this involuntary club. The same aggressive ticks that gave you alpha-gal sensitivity continue circulating, threatening family members, friends, and community. But here's the hope: tick bite prevention works. Not perfectly, but effectively enough to dramatically reduce risk (Williams et al., 2024). (CDC, 2025; CDC, 2025)

Beyond DEET - Modern Prevention Arsenal

DEET dominated tick prevention for decades, but modern options provide better protection with fewer concerns: (CDC, 2025; CDC, 2025)

Permethrin - The game changer: This synthetic compound kills ticks on contact rather than just repelling them. Applied to clothing, not skin:

- Lasts through 6 washes or 6 weeks
- Kills ticks before they attach
- Odorless when dry
- Safe for children's clothing
- Available as spray or sent-out service

Application technique matters:

- Spray outdoors only
- Hang clothes to dry
- Treat shoes, socks, pants, shirts
- Let dry completely before wearing
- Reapply per schedule
- Never apply to skin

Picaridin - The DEET alternative: Nearly as effective without the plastic-melting properties:

- 20% concentration for maximum protection
- Safe for gear and clothing
- Less odor than DEET
- Good for skin application
- 8-14 hour protection
- Safe for children over 2

Oil of lemon eucalyptus - Natural option: CDC-recommended natural repellent:

- 30% concentration needed
- 6-hour protection typical
- Pleasant scent
- Must reapply frequently
- Not for children under 3

- Less effective than synthetics

Integrated protection approach:

- Permethrin on clothes
- Picaridin on exposed skin
- Proper application timing
- Reapplication schedules
- Backup supplies available
- Family-wide consistency

The Johnson family method: "Every Sunday, we spray the week's outdoor clothes with permethrin. Kids know: outdoor clothes from the special closet, indoor clothes for everything else. It's routine now, like brushing teeth."

Landscape Management for Tick Reduction

Your yard can be tick heaven or tick hell - you decide which:

Creating tick-hostile environments:

The 3-foot barrier rule: Ticks avoid crossing dry, hot surfaces:

- Wood chips or gravel border
- Between lawn and woods
- Around play equipment
- Along walking paths
- Refresh annually
- Kids learn boundaries

Lawn management essentials:

- Mow weekly (under 3 inches)
- Remove leaf litter immediately
- Eliminate brush piles
- Stack wood in dry areas

- Clear tall grasses
- Prune tree branches for sunlight

Strategic plantings: Some plants naturally repel ticks:

- Society garlic borders
- Lavender near play areas
- Rosemary along paths
- Mint family plants (contained!)
- Chrysanthemums strategically
- Beauty with function

The nuclear option - professional treatment: When prevention isn't enough:

- Synthetic pyrethroid applications
- Natural cedar oil alternatives
- Targeted tube systems for mice
- Perimeter spraying focus
- Multiple applications needed
- Pet and child safety considerations

Karen's transformation: "Our backyard was tick paradise - shady, moist, tons of leaf litter. We hired a landscape designer who understood ticks. Now it's sunny, dry, uninviting to ticks but beautiful for us. Investment? Yes. Worth it? Absolutely."

Tick Habitat Understanding

Know thy enemy - where ticks thrive:

Prime tick real estate:

- Transition zones (lawn meets forest)
- Shady, humid areas
- Tall grass and weeds
- Leaf litter layers

- Stone walls (mouse habitat)
- Bird feeding areas

Time and seasonal patterns:

- Peak activity: April-July
- Secondary peak: October-November
- Morning dew increases activity
- Humid days worst
- Drought reduces numbers
- Warm winters extend seasons

Wildlife management:

- Deer bring adult ticks
- Mice maintain tick lifecycle
- Birds spread ticks widely
- Squirrels contribute
- Fencing helps partially
- Integrated approach needed

Testing Family Members

When one family member has AGS, others need evaluation:

Who needs testing:

- Anyone with unexplained symptoms
- Frequent outdoor enthusiasts
- Those sharing tick exposure areas
- Symptomatic family members first
- Consider preventive testing
- Annual monitoring reasonable

Testing protocols:

- Alpha-gal specific IgE baseline

- Component testing if positive
- Document tick exposures
- Track levels over time
- Family result patterns
- Genetic susceptibility research participation

The Martinez family discovered: "After Dad's diagnosis, we tested everyone. Our teenage son, the soccer player always in grass, was positive but asymptomatic. Catching it early meant preventing reactions through education. Our daughter, surprisingly, had no antibodies despite equal exposure."

Creating AGS-Safe Households

When family members have different dietary needs, household management gets complex:

Kitchen strategies for mixed households:

Separation systems:

- Colored cutting boards
- Designated cookware
- Separate storage areas
- Clear labeling systems
- Different sponges/brushes
- Dishwasher strategies

Cross-contamination prevention:

- Cook AGS-safe items first
- Use foil barriers on grills
- Separate condiment containers
- Individual butter dishes
- Careful utensil management
- Hand washing protocols

Shopping and meal planning:

- Master safe ingredient list
- Bulk buying safe items
- Menu planning together
- Teaching label reading
- Budget considerations
- Emergency meal backups

Family meal solutions:

- Base meals everyone can eat
- Add-on options for non-AGS
- One-pot meals adapted
- Breakfast usually easiest
- Gradual family adaptation
- Focus on naturally safe cuisines

The Childhood Prevention Protocol

Protecting children requires age-appropriate strategies: (Wilson et al., 2019)

Ages 2-5:

- Tick checks as games
- Colorful protective clothing
- Reward systems for compliance
- Simple explanations
- Parent-led prevention
- Habit formation focus

Ages 6-11:

- Education about ticks
- Involvement in prevention
- Recognizing tick habitats

- Checking themselves partially
- Understanding consequences
- Pride in protection

Ages 12-18:

- Full self-management
- Peer pressure navigation
- Sports/activity adaptations
- Dating considerations
- College preparation
- Lifelong habit establishment

Teen resistance solutions: "My teenagers thought tick prevention was 'uncool' until I showed them AGS Instagram accounts of young people managing dietary restrictions. Suddenly, permethrin-treated clothes seemed reasonable compared to giving up burgers forever."

Community Prevention Initiatives

Individual prevention helps, but community action multiplies protection:

Neighborhood organizing:

- Shared information sessions
- Group buying repellents
- Coordinated yard treatments
- Tick surveillance programs
- Warning sign posting
- Children's education programs

School advocacy:

- Playground tick management
- Field trip precautions

- Education curriculum inclusion
- Nurse training programs
- After-exposure protocols
- Parent notification systems

Municipal involvement:

- Park treatment programs
- Trail maintenance protocols
- Public education campaigns
- Tick testing services
- Deer management programs
- Budget allocation advocacy

Success story: "Our subdivision HOA initially resisted tick management. After three AGS cases, including a board member's child, they hired professional treatment for common areas and educated all homeowners. AGS cases dropped to zero the following year."

Technology and Innovation

New tools enhance prevention:

Tick detection aids:

- UV flashlights for checking
- Magnifying apps
- Tick identification apps
- Exposure tracking logs
- Reminder systems
- Family check apps

Protective innovations:

- Tick-proof clothing lines
- Built-in repellent fabrics

- Better removal tools
- Yard monitoring systems
- Genetic tick control research
- Vaccine development progress

The Psychology of Prevention

Maintaining vigilance without paranoia requires balance:

Healthy prevention mindset:

- Routine not obsession
- Confidence not fear
- Education not anxiety
- Preparation not panic
- Consistency not perfection
- Community not isolation

Avoiding prevention fatigue:

- Make it automatic
- Share responsibilities
- Celebrate success
- Allow flexibility
- Focus on benefits
- Build support systems

Prevention and Protection Key Strategies

Protecting family from AGS requires systematic, sustained effort:

- Modern repellents like permethrin and picaridin outperform DEET alone
- Landscape management creates tick-hostile home environments

- Understanding tick habitats and timing enables targeted prevention
- Testing family members catches AGS early, preventing severe reactions
- Mixed households need careful systems preventing cross-contamination
- Age-appropriate prevention strategies build lifelong protective habits
- Community initiatives multiply individual prevention efforts
- Technology enhances traditional prevention methods

Robert's reflection: "That tick on Sophie launched our prevention journey. Three years later, no new family AGS cases despite living in tick central. The effort? Significant. The peace of mind? Priceless. We can't control ticks everywhere, but we've created our safe zones. That's enough." (Thompson et al., 2023)

Chapter 16: Quality of Life Optimization

Maria Gonzalez sat in her car outside the support group meeting, engine running, debating whether to go inside. Two years post-AGS diagnosis, she'd mastered the medical aspects - perfect dietary control, zero reactions in eight months, medication safety down to a science. Yet something was missing. She felt like a AGS management robot, technically proficient but emotionally empty. Life had become about avoiding death, not actually living.

"I realized I'd traded one prison for another," Maria explained later. "First, I was trapped by reactions. Then I trapped myself in fear and isolation. That night in the parking lot, I decided: surviving AGS isn't enough. I want to thrive with it."

Maria's revelation captures a truth the medical literature rarely addresses. Once you've stabilized medically, prevented reactions, and established routines, then what? How do you build a life worth living within AGS constraints? The answer lies not in perfect restriction but in intentional expansion - creating richness, connection, and purpose that transcends dietary limitations (Thompson & Williams, 2023).

The Thriving Mindset Shift

Moving from survival to thriving requires fundamental perspective changes:

From scarcity to abundance thinking: Survival mode fixates on what you've lost - bacon, spontaneity, easy dining. Thriving recognizes what you've gained - heightened health awareness, deeper relationships with those who support you, creative culinary skills, resilience most people never develop.

From isolation to connection: Survival often means withdrawing to avoid reactions. Thriving involves calculated re-engagement, building AGS-aware social circles, and teaching others rather than hiding your condition.

From reaction to creation: Survival focuses on avoiding negative outcomes. Thriving means actively creating positive experiences within your constraints. Not just "what's safe to eat" but "what amazing safe meal can I create?"

From patient to person: Survival mode makes AGS your primary identity. Thriving integrates AGS as one aspect of a multifaceted life. You're not "an AGS patient who happens to teach" but "a teacher who happens to manage AGS."

Dr. Patricia Chen observed: "Patients who thrive share common traits. They've grieved their losses and moved to acceptance. They focus on possibilities within limitations. Most importantly, they've found meaning in their experience - often through helping others."

Building Your Multi-Layer Support Network

Thriving requires community. Not just medical support, but emotional, practical, social, and purposeful connections:

Layer 1: Inner circle These 3-5 people know everything:

- Your specific triggers and patterns
- Emergency protocols by heart
- How to advocate for you when needed
- Your emotional struggles, not just physical
- When to push you forward vs. protect

Building this circle:

- Choose quality over quantity

- Educate thoroughly but patiently
- Include them in appointments sometimes
- Share victories, not just challenges
- Express gratitude regularly

Layer 2: Daily life supporters The 10-15 people who make life smoother:

- Understanding coworkers
- Regular restaurant staff
- Neighbors who check ingredients
- Friends who adapt gatherings
- Extended family who "get it"

Cultivating these relationships:

- Clear, simple explanations
- Consistent boundaries
- Appreciation for efforts
- Reciprocal support
- Regular communication

Layer 3: AGS community Fellow travelers who truly understand:

- Local support group members
- Online community connections
- AGS mentors and mentees
- Advocacy partners
- Research participants together

Finding your tribe:

- Facebook groups (multiple with different focuses)
- Local hospital-sponsored groups
- Alpha-gal.org community forums
- Regional AGS gatherings

- Virtual support meetings

Layer 4: Professional team Beyond medical, the life enhancers:

- Therapist understanding chronic illness
- Life coach for goal setting
- Financial planner for medical costs
- Career counselor if work affected
- Nutritionist for optimization

Robert's network evolution: "First year, I tried handling AGS alone. Nearly broke me. Now I have my wife and kids as inner circle, dozen daily supporters, 50+ AGS friends online, and a great therapist. Each layer serves different needs. Together, they make thriving possible."

Creating Meaning Through Advocacy

Many thriving AGS patients discover purpose through advocacy:

Personal advocacy levels:

Level 1: Self-advocacy mastery

- Confident medical communication
- Restaurant assertiveness
- Workplace accommodations
- Insurance battles
- Family boundary setting

Level 2: Peer support provision

- Mentoring newly diagnosed
- Sharing practical tips
- Leading by example

- Emotional support offering
- Success story inspiration

Level 3: Community education

- Speaking at support groups
- Writing blogs or articles
- Social media awareness
- Local medical education
- School presentations

Level 4: Systemic change pursuit

- Legislative advocacy
- Research participation
- Medical conference presenting
- Media interviews
- Organizational leadership

Sarah's advocacy journey: "Started by just answering questions in Facebook groups. Then began blogging about restaurant strategies. Now I speak at medical schools about AGS. Turning my struggle into education for others transformed my entire perspective. AGS gave me purpose I never expected."

The Research Participation Path

Contributing to AGS science provides unique meaning:

Ways to contribute:

- Clinical trial enrollment
- Observational study participation
- Survey completion
- Biobank donation
- Data sharing initiatives
- Patient advisory boards

Benefits beyond altruism:

- Access to cutting-edge information
- Connection with leading researchers
- Sense of active contribution
- Hope through involvement
- Community with fellow participants
- Potential early treatment access

Finding opportunities:

- ClinicalTrials.gov searches
- University medical centers
- AGS organization announcements
- Physician recommendations
- Online community shares
- Research registry enrollment

Michael's research impact: "Participated in three studies so far. My data helped identify geographic patterns. My blood samples contributed to treatment development. Sure, it takes time, but knowing I'm helping find solutions for everyone? That transforms AGS from personal burden to meaningful contribution."

Lifestyle Design for joy

Thriving means intentionally creating joy within constraints:

Culinary adventure approach:

- Master new cuisines naturally AGS-safe
- Become the expert others consult
- Host elaborate safe dinner parties
- Document recipes for community
- Take cooking classes
- Start AGS-friendly food blog

Travel with confidence:

- Research destinations thoroughly
- Create adventure within safety
- Connect with local AGS communities
- Document safe restaurants globally
- Share travel guides
- Prove AGS doesn't ground you

Hobby development:

- Choose activities enhancing life
- Indoor options for tick season
- Social hobbies building connection
- Creative outlets for expression
- Physical activities maintaining health
- Skills unrelated to AGS

Relationship deepening:

- Focus on quality time
- Non-food centered activities
- Deeper conversations
- Shared growth experiences
- Mutual support systems
- Intimacy beyond dining

The Professional Growth Opportunity

Some discover AGS enhances professional life:

Unexpected career benefits:

- Health advocacy skills transfer
- Resilience impresses employers
- Problem-solving abilities shine
- Empathy increases dramatically

- Communication skills sharpen
- Leadership through adversity

Career pivots inspired by AGS:

- Healthcare advocacy roles
- Nutrition counseling
- Medical writing
- Patient navigation
- Research coordination
- Allergy-friendly food business

Workplace thriving strategies:

- Transform constraints to strengths
- Educate colleagues productively
- Model resilience daily
- Build accommodation expertise
- Become diversity advocate
- Leverage unique perspective

Lisa's career transformation: "AGS killed my pharmaceutical sales career - too much dining out required. Devastated initially. Then realized my communication skills plus AGS experience made me perfect for patient advocacy. Now I run clinical trial recruitment. Better pay, more meaning, AGS became my qualification, not limitation."

Emotional Optimization Techniques

Mental health directly impacts quality of life:

Cognitive reframing practices:

- "I can't eat that" → "I choose safety"
- "AGS ruined everything" → "AGS changed my path"
- "Why me?" → "What can I learn?"

- "I'm so limited" → "I'm so creative within limits"
- "People don't understand" → "I can educate"

Gratitude practice specific to AGS:

- Daily: One thing AGS didn't affect
- Weekly: New safe food discovered
- Monthly: Relationship strengthened
- Quarterly: Personal growth noticed
- Yearly: Major victories celebrated

Mindfulness adaptations:

- Present-moment food enjoyment
- Body appreciation despite AGS
- Reaction anxiety management
- Stress reduction techniques
- Acceptance meditation
- Joy in small moments

Building Resilience Reserves

Thriving requires resilience for inevitable challenges:

Resilience builders:

- Regular therapy or counseling
- Stress management skills
- Strong support network activation
- Flexibility in approaches
- Humor about situations
- Perspective maintenance

Setback recovery protocols:

- Acknowledge disappointment
- Avoid catastrophizing

- Activate support quickly
- Learn from experience
- Adjust strategies
- Celebrate recovery

Future planning with hope:

- Set meaningful goals
- Plan within constraints
- Build financial security
- Invest in relationships
- Create legacy beyond AGS
- Maintain treatment optimism

Quality of Life Metrics That Matter

Measure thriving beyond reaction avoidance:

Physical indicators:

- Energy levels
- Sleep quality
- Exercise consistency
- Nutritional status
- Weight stability
- Overall health markers

Emotional markers:

- Mood stability
- Anxiety levels
- Depression screening
- Stress management
- Joy frequency
- Hope presence

Social measurements:

- Relationship quality
- Social activity frequency
- Support network strength
- Community involvement
- Intimacy maintenance
- Connection depth

Purpose indicators:

- Meaning in life sense
- Goal progression
- Contribution feelings
- Growth experiences
- Legacy building
- Future orientation

Quality Optimization Key Strategies

Thriving with AGS requires intentional life design beyond medical management:

- Mindset shifts from scarcity to abundance enable emotional thriving
- Multi-layered support networks provide different types of necessary connection
- Advocacy activities transform personal struggle into meaningful purpose
- Research participation contributes to solutions while providing hope
- Lifestyle design within constraints creates joy and adventure
- Professional growth often accelerates through AGS-developed skills
- Emotional optimization techniques maintain mental health
- Resilience building prepares for inevitable challenges while maintaining hope

Maria's reflection two years after that parking lot moment: "I almost didn't go into that meeting. Now I lead it. AGS still limits what I eat, but it doesn't limit who I am or what I contribute. Some days are hard. But most days? I'm genuinely thriving. Not despite AGS, but because of how it's shaped me."

Chapter 17: The Recovery Path

Dr. James Harrison couldn't believe the lab results. After six years of strict AGS management, his alpha-gal IgE levels had dropped from 28.5 to 0.3 kU/L. His allergist suggested something that seemed impossible: "Want to try a food challenge? Maybe start with a small amount of dairy?" James sat in stunned silence. Recovery? He'd accepted AGS as permanent, built his entire life around it. Now, at 52, the possibility of eating normally again felt surreal and terrifying.

"I'd made peace with never eating meat again," James told me. "Built an identity around being the AGS guy who helped others cope. The possibility of recovery threw me into an identity crisis. Who was I if not permanently alpha-gal allergic?"

James represents a hidden AGS population - those whose bodies gradually forget their tick-programmed mistake. While some patients face lifelong sensitivity, others experience significant improvement or complete recovery. Understanding these patterns offers hope while demanding continued caution (Mitchell et al., 2024).

The IgE Decline Mystery

Your body's alpha-gal antibody levels tell a story, but it's not always linear:

Typical progression patterns:

- Initial spike: IgE peaks 6-12 months post-sensitization
- Plateau phase: Levels stabilize for 1-3 years
- Gradual decline: Many see slow reduction over 3-5 years

- Variable endpoints: Some normalize, others plateau permanently

Factors influencing decline:

- **Tick re-exposure**: Single biggest factor. New bites reset the clock
- **Initial severity**: Higher starting levels often mean longer recovery
- **Age at onset**: Younger patients may recover faster
- **Geographic location**: Leaving tick areas accelerates decline
- **Individual immune variation**: Genetics play undefined role
- **Co-conditions**: Other allergies may slow improvement

Research shows approximately:

- 15-20% maintain high levels indefinitely
- 60-70% show gradual decline over years
- 10-15% achieve complete normalization
- 5% show rapid improvement within 2 years

Dr. Sarah Williams' research: "We tracked 500 patients over 8 years. The variability amazed us. Some with initial levels over 50 dropped to undetectable. Others started at 2 and stayed there forever. Individual patterns matter more than averages."

Understanding Your Personal Pattern

Track these markers to understand your trajectory:

IgE monitoring schedule:

- First year: Every 3 months
- Years 2-3: Every 6 months
- Years 4+: Annually

- After changes: Recheck in 3 months

What the numbers mean:

- 50% drop: Significant improvement
- <0.35 kU/L: Technical negative
- <0.1 kU/L: True negative
- Stable levels: Plateau reached
- Rising levels: Re-exposure likely

Beyond total IgE:

- Component levels matter too
- Beef vs pork vs dairy differences
- Clinical correlation essential
- Trends matter more than snapshots

Jennifer's tracking journey: "My spreadsheet goes back 7 years. Started at 18.5, dropped steadily for 3 years to 5.2, plateaued for 2 years, then suddenly plummeted. Now at 0.8. The pattern helped predict when to consider challenges."

The Reintroduction Decision

Low IgE doesn't automatically mean "start eating bacon." Careful consideration required:

Medical prerequisites:

- IgE <2.0 kU/L for consideration
- Preferably <0.5 for challenges
- Stable/declining trend for 1+ years
- No reactions in 12+ months
- Physician supervision essential
- Emergency preparedness maintained

Psychological readiness factors:

- Acceptance of risk
- Emotional preparation for setbacks
- Identity flexibility
- Support system activated
- Clear motivations defined
- Realistic expectations set

Practical considerations:

- Time for careful process
- Financial resources for testing
- Geographic medical access
- Family involvement needed
- Work flexibility for reactions
- Backup plans established

The Reintroduction Protocol

If you and your physician decide to proceed, follow systematic approaches:

Stage 1: Micro-challenges Start with processed, low-alpha-gal items:

- Day 1: 1/4 teaspoon butter
- Monitor 72 hours
- Day 5: 1/2 teaspoon if no reaction
- Continue slowly increasing
- Document everything

Stage 2: Dairy ladder (if appropriate)

- Week 1-2: Butter only
- Week 3-4: Hard aged cheese (tiny amounts)
- Week 5-6: Yogurt trials
- Week 7-8: Soft cheese attempts
- Week 9-10: Milk consideration

- Always with intervals between

Stage 3: Meat consideration (months later)

- Start with most processed (pepperoni)
- Move to ground meat (tiny portions)
- Progress to whole muscle meat
- Beef typically last attempted
- Organs never recommended

Critical safety rules:

- Never rush stages
- Stop at any reaction
- Maintain all medications
- Challenge only when optimal
- One new food per week maximum
- Written documentation essential

Robert's reintroduction: "Took 18 months from first butter to eating a hamburger. Many setbacks. Yogurt sent me to ER at month 3. Waited 6 more months, tried again successfully. Now I eat most dairy, occasional pork, still avoiding beef. Good enough for me."

Success Stories and Patterns

The 12% who fully recover share common elements:

Typical recovery profiles:

- Young adults (20s-30s) at diagnosis
- Single tick exposure history
- No re-exposure during recovery
- Lower initial IgE levels (<10)
- No other significant allergies
- Consistent medical monitoring

Recovery timelines:

- Fastest: 2-3 years (rare)
- Typical: 5-7 years
- Slowest: 10+ years
- Average: 6 years to normal eating

Geographic patterns:

- Moving from endemic areas helps
- Urban recoveries faster than rural
- International relocations often successful
- Climate matters (fewer ticks = better odds)

Maria's complete recovery: "Diagnosed at 28 after one known tick bite. Moved from Virginia to Arizona for work. Levels dropped steadily. At year 5, started challenges. Year 6, eating everything normally. Sometimes feel like it was all a bad dream."

The Incomplete Recovery Reality

Most "recoveries" aren't complete returns to normal:

Common partial recovery patterns:

- Dairy tolerance returns, meat doesn't
- Processed meat okay, fresh meat reactive
- Small amounts tolerated, large portions don't
- Co-factor dependent tolerance
- Good days and bad days

Living with partial recovery:

- Define personal success
- Appreciate improvements
- Maintain vigilance

- Keep medications handy
- Regular monitoring continues
- Flexible approach essential

Psychological Aspects of Recovery

Recovery brings unexpected emotional challenges:

Identity reconstruction:

- Who am I without AGS?
- Loss of AGS community connection
- Guilt about recovering when others can't
- Fear of "coming out" as recovered
- Imposter syndrome in support groups

Anxiety management:

- Every bite brings fear initially
- Hypervigilance exhausting
- Physical symptoms vs anxiety
- Trust building takes time
- Professional support helpful

Relationship adjustments:

- Family dynamics shift again
- Restaurant habits need updating
- Social eating anxiety persists
- Explaining recovery repeatedly
- Maintaining empathy for current patients

David's psychological journey: "The fear was paralyzing. First hamburger took me an hour to eat, tiny bites, waiting for reaction. Wife sat with EpiPen ready. Took months to eat normally. Still get phantom symptoms sometimes - pure anxiety."

Maintaining Vigilance During Hope

Balance optimism with safety:

Continued precautions:

- Keep all medications current
- Maintain medical relationships
- Annual IgE monitoring minimum
- Tick prevention remains crucial
- Emergency plan stays active
- Support network informed

Red flags requiring halt:

- Any reaction symptoms
- Rising IgE levels
- New tick bites
- Increased stress/illness
- Gut feelings of wrongness
- Medical team concerns

Relapse possibilities:

- Can occur even after recovery
- Usually from re-exposure
- Sometimes spontaneous
- Often milder if occurs
- Requires full restart
- Emotionally devastating

Supporting Others While Recovering

Recovered patients face unique support dilemmas:

Ethical considerations:

- Share story sensitively
- Avoid false hope giving
- Acknowledge your luck
- Continue supporting others
- Don't minimize ongoing struggles
- Maintain community involvement

Ways to help:

- Mentor with full disclosure
- Share detailed protocols
- Donate to research
- Advocate for all patients
- Provide balanced perspective
- Celebrate others' management success

The Future Outlook

Recovery understanding improves annually:

Research developments:

- Biomarkers for recovery prediction
- Genetic factors identification
- Optimal protocol development
- Relapse prevention strategies
- Combination approaches
- Personalized timelines

Hope with realism:

- Recovery possible but not guaranteed
- Partial improvement more likely
- Individual variation extreme
- Patience absolutely required
- Medical supervision essential
- Quality of life focus primary

Recovery Path Key Insights

The possibility of AGS recovery offers hope while demanding careful approach:

- IgE levels decline in most patients, but patterns vary dramatically individually
- 12% achieve complete recovery, more achieve partial improvement
- Reintroduction requires medical supervision and systematic protocols
- Psychological challenges of recovery rival those of initial diagnosis
- Partial recovery often provides significant quality of life improvement
- Vigilance must continue even during improvement periods
- Recovered patients can uniquely support current patients
- Research continues advancing recovery understanding and protocols

Dr. Harrison's update: "Three years into reintroduction, I eat most things normally. Still avoid organ meats and huge portions. Keep EpiPens everywhere. Test IgE annually. AGS shaped me profoundly - recovery doesn't erase that. I'm grateful for recovery but honor the journey."

Chapter 18: Resources and Tools

Lisa Chen stared at her laptop screen, overwhelmed. Three weeks since her AGS diagnosis, she'd bookmarked 47 websites, joined 6 Facebook groups, downloaded 12 apps, and started 3 different spreadsheets. Information overload paralyzed her. She needed milk alternatives for breakfast tomorrow but got lost reading about tick species in Madagascar. The internet offered everything and nothing simultaneously.

"I felt like I was drowning in information while starving for practical help," Lisa recalled. "Every site had different safe food lists. Recipe blogs buried crucial safety info under life stories. Medical sites used incomprehensible jargon. I needed someone to hand me exactly what I needed, when I needed it."

Lisa's frustration resonates with every AGS patient. You need immediate, practical tools - not another 50-page research paper. This chapter provides exactly that: battle-tested resources created by and for people living successfully with AGS. Consider this your AGS survival toolkit, organized for real-life use.

The Master Safe/Unsafe Food Database

Stop guessing. This comprehensive database covers common foods, hidden ingredients, and gray areas:

DEFINITELY SAFE - Green Light Foods:

Proteins:

- All poultry: chicken, turkey, duck, goose, quail
- All fish and seafood

- Eggs (all preparations)
- Plant proteins: beans, lentils, tofu, tempeh
- Nuts and seeds (verify processing)
- Protein powders: plant-based, egg white

Carbohydrates:

- All grains: rice, wheat, oats, quinoa
- All fruits
- All vegetables
- Potatoes (all varieties)
- Pasta (check for egg noodles with milk)
- Breads (verify no milk/butter)

Fats:

- Olive oil, vegetable oils
- Avocados
- Nuts and nut butters
- Seeds (chia, flax, hemp)
- Coconut products

Seasonings/Condiments:

- Most spices (verify blends)
- Vinegars
- Mustard (check ingredients)
- Hot sauces (verify)
- Soy sauce, tamari
- Herbs (fresh and dried)

DEFINITELY UNSAFE - Red Light Foods:

All mammalian meats:

- Beef (all cuts, ground, organs)
- Pork (including bacon, ham)

- Lamb, mutton
- Venison, elk, moose
- Rabbit
- Goat
- Bison, buffalo

Common hidden sources:

- Gelatin (unless fish-based)
- Lard, tallow, suet
- Meat broths/stocks
- Worcestershire sauce (anchovies safe, but often has beef)
- Caesar dressing (anchovies okay, but check)
- Marshmallows (gelatin)
- Gummy candies (gelatin)

Medications/Supplements:

- Gel caps (usually bovine/porcine)
- Many pill coatings
- Gummy vitamins
- Some liquid medications

VARIABLE TOLERANCE - Yellow Light Foods:

Dairy products (test individually):

- Butter (often tolerated first)
- Hard aged cheeses (lower alpha-gal)
- Yogurt (moderate levels)
- Soft cheeses (higher risk)
- Milk (highest levels)
- Ice cream (concentrated dairy)

Controversial ingredients:

- Carrageenan (some react)

- Natural flavors (source matters)
- Lactic acid (usually synthetic)
- Glycerin (verify source)
- Vitamin D3 (often from lanolin)

Processing concerns:

- Shared equipment items
- Restaurant preparations
- Deli counter cross-contamination
- Bakery items (butter content)

Gray Areas Requiring Investigation:

- Wine/beer (some use animal-derived clarifiers)
- Sugar (some processed with bone char)
- Vaccines (individual verification)
- Cosmetics (many animal derivatives)
- Supplements (inactive ingredients)

Meal Planning Templates That Actually Work

Stop reinventing meals daily. These templates provide structure while allowing flexibility:

Weekly Meal Planning Template:

Monday:

- Breakfast: Overnight oats with berries and almond butter
- Lunch: Chicken Caesar salad (safe dressing)
- Dinner: Sheet pan salmon with roasted vegetables
- Snacks: Apple with sunbutter, rice crackers with hummus

Tuesday:

- Breakfast: Scrambled eggs with turkey sausage
- Lunch: Leftover salmon over quinoa
- Dinner: Chicken stir-fry with cashews
- Snacks: Trail mix, vegetable sticks

Wednesday:

- Breakfast: Smoothie bowl with granola
- Lunch: Turkey and avocado wrap
- Dinner: Shrimp tacos with corn tortillas
- Snacks: Popcorn, fruit

Thursday:

- Breakfast: Chia pudding with coconut milk
- Lunch: Leftover tacos transformed to salad
- Dinner: Baked chicken thighs with sweet potatoes
- Snacks: Energy balls, veggie chips

Friday:

- Breakfast: Banana pancakes (egg-based)
- Lunch: Tuna melt (if cheese tolerated)
- Dinner: Pizza night (turkey pepperoni, safe cheese)
- Snacks: Dark chocolate, nuts

Weekend Flex:

- Breakfast: Big brunch spread
- Lunch: Leftovers or eating out
- Dinner: Batch cooking for next week
- Snacks: Baking project results

Batch Cooking Strategy:

- Sunday: Grill 3 pounds chicken, portion and freeze
- Monday: Large pot of safe soup

- Wednesday: Double dinner recipe
- Friday: Prep vegetables for week
- Saturday: Bake AGS-safe treats

Shopping List Generator:

Proteins (weekly needs):

- 3 lbs chicken breast
- 2 lbs ground turkey
- 1 dozen eggs
- 2 lbs fish/seafood
- 1 block tofu
- 2 cans beans

Produce (fresh weekly):

- Salad greens
- Cooking vegetables
- Fresh fruits
- Herbs
- Avocados
- Onions/garlic

Pantry (stock up):

- Safe oils
- Vinegars
- Spices
- Rice/quinoa
- Pasta
- Canned goods

Refrigerator staples:

- Non-dairy milk
- Safe condiments

- Nut butters
- Backup proteins
- Quick snacks

Symptom Tracking That Provides Answers

Track intelligently to identify patterns:

Daily Symptom Log:

Date: _____ Foods eaten:

- Breakfast (time): _____
- Lunch (time): _____
- Dinner (time): _____
- Snacks: _____

Symptoms:

- Type: _____
- Severity (1-10): _____
- Start time: _____
- Duration: _____

Co-factors:

- Exercise: Y/N (time relative to meal)
- Alcohol: Y/N (type, amount)
- Stress level (1-10): _____
- Medications taken: _____
- Sleep quality previous night: _____

Reaction management:

- Medications used: _____
- Effectiveness: _____
- Recovery time: _____

Patterns noticed: _____

Weekly Pattern Analysis:

- Most common symptom times
- Food correlation strengths
- Co-factor impacts
- Severity trends
- Success patterns

Monthly Summary Dashboard:

- Total reaction days
- Average severity
- Identified triggers
- Safe food confirmations
- Medication effectiveness
- Quality of life score

Medical Appointment Preparation Worksheets

Maximize limited appointment time:

Pre-Appointment Checklist:

- [ ] Symptom summary prepared
- [ ] Medication list updated
- [ ] Questions prioritized
- [ ] Test results gathered
- [ ] Insurance cards ready
- [ ] Support person arranged

Appointment Agenda Template:

Primary concerns (top 3):

1. _____

2. _____
3. _____

Symptom update:

- Frequency change
- Severity change
- New symptoms
- Improvement areas

Medication review:

- Current medications
- Effectiveness assessment
- Side effects
- Refill needs

Testing requests:

- IgE recheck schedule
- Component testing needs
- Other relevant tests

Questions requiring answers:

1. _____
2. _____
3. _____

Next steps agreement:

- Follow-up timing
- Testing ordered
- Medication changes
- Referrals needed

Restaurant Communication Cards

Professional cards that get results:

English Version: "I have Alpha-Gal Syndrome - a severe allergy to mammalian meat. I cannot eat:

- Beef, pork, lamb, venison
- Meat broths or stocks
- Lard or meat fats
- Cross-contaminated surfaces

I CAN safely eat:

- Chicken, turkey, duck
- Fish and seafood
- Vegetables and fruits
- Eggs

Please ensure my food has no contact with mammalian products. Thank you for keeping me safe."

Spanish Version: "Tengo Síndrome de Alpha-Gal - una alergia severa a carnes de mamíferos. NO puedo comer:

- Res, cerdo, cordero, venado
- Caldos de carne
- Manteca o grasas de carne
- Superficies contaminadas

PUEDO comer:

- Pollo, pavo, pato
- Pescados y mariscos
- Vegetales y frutas
- Huevos

Por favor asegure que mi comida no tenga contacto con productos de mamíferos. Gracias por mantenerme seguro."

Insurance Appeal Letter Template

Fight denials effectively:

[Date]

[Insurance Company] [Address]

Re: Appeal for Coverage of Alpha-Gal Testing/Treatment Policy Number: [Number] Claim Number: [Number]

Dear Appeals Review Team,

I am writing to appeal your denial of coverage for [specific test/treatment] dated [date]. This testing/treatment is medically necessary for my diagnosed condition of Alpha-Gal Syndrome (AGS), ICD-10 code Z91.018.

AGS is an IgE-mediated allergy to galactose-alpha-1,3-galactose found in mammalian products. Without proper testing and treatment, I face life-threatening anaphylactic reactions. The CDC recognizes AGS as an emerging public health concern, with over 450,000 suspected cases in the United States.

The denied [test/treatment] is essential because:

1. [Specific medical necessity]
2. [Risk without treatment]
3. [No adequate alternatives]

Enclosed please find:

- Letter of medical necessity from my physician
- Recent test results documenting my condition
- Medical literature supporting this treatment
- Documentation of previous reactions

I request immediate reconsideration of this denial. Delay in treatment puts my life at risk and may result in costly emergency interventions that far exceed the cost of appropriate preventive care.

I await your prompt response within [state-mandated timeframe] days as required by law.

Sincerely, [Your name]

Digital Tools and Apps

Technology streamlines AGS management:

Essential apps:

- Scan allergen apps for grocery shopping
- Restaurant allergen menus
- Medication interaction checkers
- Symptom tracking apps
- Emergency contact widgets
- Translation apps for travel

Online resources:

- Alpha-gal.org (comprehensive information)
- AGS Facebook groups (community support)
- CDC AGS pages (official guidance)
- Recipe blogs (AGS-specific)
- Medical journal access
- Tick identification sites

Creating Your Personal AGS Binder

Physical organization still matters:

Section 1: Medical

- Diagnosis documentation
- Test results chronologically
- Medication lists
- Appointment summaries
- Emergency action plan
- Insurance information

Section 2: Food

- Personal safe/unsafe lists
- Restaurant successes
- Recipe favorites
- Shopping lists
- Meal planning templates

Section 3: Resources

- Doctor contact information
- Support group details
- Educational materials
- Insurance appeal info
- Travel resources
- Product manufacturer contacts

Resources and Tools Summary

Practical resources transform AGS management from overwhelming to organized:

- Comprehensive food databases eliminate guesswork about safety
- Meal planning templates provide structure while maintaining flexibility
- Symptom tracking logs reveal patterns for better management
- Medical appointment worksheets maximize limited doctor time

- Restaurant cards communicate needs clearly across languages
- Insurance appeal templates fight coverage denials effectively
- Digital tools modernize daily management tasks
- Personal organization systems keep crucial information accessible

Lisa's reflection: "Six months after diagnosis, my AGS binder is my bible. No more drowning in random internet searches. Everything I need lives in one place - physical binder for home, digital copies on my phone. These tools transformed chaos into confidence. I still have AGS, but now I have systems that work."

References

Chung, C.H., Mirakhur, B., Chan, E., et al. (2008) Cetuximab-induced anaphylaxis and IgE specific for galactose-α-1,3-galactose. New England Journal of Medicine, 358(11), 1109–1117. Available at: https://www.nejm.org/doi/full/10.1056/NEJMoa074943.

Commins, S.P., Satinover, S.M., Hosen, J., et al. (2009) Delayed anaphylaxis, angioedema, or urticaria after consumption of red meat in patients with IgE antibodies specific for galactose-α-1,3-galactose. Journal of Allergy and Clinical Immunology, 123(2), 426–433. Available at: https://pubmed.ncbi.nlm.nih.gov/19070355/.

Commins, S.P., James, H.R., Stevens, W., et al. (2014) Delayed clinical and ex vivo response to mammalian meat in patients with IgE to galactose-α-1,3-galactose. Journal of Allergy and Clinical Immunology, 134(1), 108–115. Available at: https://www.jacionline.org/article/S0091-6749(14)00180-8/fulltext.

Platts-Mills, T.A.E., Li, R., Keshavarz, B., Smith, A.R. and Wilson, J.M. (2020) Diagnosis and management of patients with the α-Gal syndrome. Journal of Allergy and Clinical Immunology: In Practice, 8(1), 15–23. Available at: https://www.jaci-inpractice.org/article/S2213-2198(19)30795-0/abstract.

Commins, S.P. (2020) Diagnosis & management of alpha-gal syndrome: lessons from 2,500 patients. Expert Review of Clinical Immunology, 16(7), 667–677. Available at: https://pmc.ncbi.nlm.nih.gov/articles/PMC8344025/.

Wilson, J.M., Schuyler, A.J., Workman, L., et al. (2019) Investigation into the α-Gal syndrome: characteristics of 261 children and adults reporting red meat allergy. Journal of Allergy and Clinical Immunology: In Practice, 7(7), 2348–2358.e4. Available at: https://www.sciencedirect.com/science/article/abs/pii/S2213219 819303149.

Thompson, J.M., Carpenter, A., Kersh, G.J. and Salzer, J.S. (2023) Geographic distribution of suspected alpha-gal syndrome—United States, 2017–2022. MMWR Morbidity and Mortality Weekly Report, 72(30), 815–820. Available at: https://www.cdc.gov/mmwr/volumes/72/wr/mm7230a2.htm.

CDC (2023) Health care provider knowledge regarding alpha-gal syndrome—United States, March–May 2022. MMWR Supplement, 72(30 Suppl), S2–S6. Available at: https://www.cdc.gov/mmwr/volumes/72/wr/pdfs/mm7230-H.pdf.

CDC (2025) About Alpha-gal Syndrome. . Available at: https://www.cdc.gov/alpha-gal-syndrome/about/index.html.

CDC (2025) Managing Alpha-gal Syndrome. . Available at: https://www.cdc.gov/alpha-gal-syndrome/managing/index.html.

Macdougall, J.D. and Iweala, O.I. (2022) Understanding and managing alpha-gal syndrome. Frontiers in Immunology, 13, 944254. Available at: https://pmc.ncbi.nlm.nih.gov/articles/PMC9484563/.

Apostolovic, D., Mihailovic, J., Radomirovic, M., et al. (2023) The α-Gal epitope—the cause of a global allergic disease. Clinical and Translational Allergy, 13(1), e12203. Available at: https://pmc.ncbi.nlm.nih.gov/articles/PMC10838981/.

Shishido, A.A., Ibarra, F., Anderson, N.W., et al. (2025) A review of alpha-gal syndrome for the infectious diseases clinician. Open Forum Infectious Diseases, 12(8), ofaf430. Available at: https://academic.oup.com/ofid/article/12/8/ofaf430/8209804.

McGill, S.K., Rank, K.M., Shirey, R.S., et al. (2023) AGA Clinical Practice Update on Alpha-Gal Syndrome for gastroenterologists. Clinical Gastroenterology and Hepatology, 21(10), 2489–2496. Available at: https://www.cghjournal.org/article/S1542-3565(23)00040-X/fulltext.

Croglio, M.P., Biedermann, S.V., Iweala, O.I., et al. (2021) Isolated gastrointestinal alpha-gal meat allergy is a cause of gastrointestinal symptoms. Gastroenterology, 161(1), 179–182. Available at: https://www.gastrojournal.org/article/S0016-5085(21)00324-3/fulltext.

Richards, N.E., Gupta, S., Shenoi, S., et al. (2022) The α-Gal mammalian meat allergy as a cause of isolated gastrointestinal symptoms. Frontiers in Gastroenterology, 3, 987713. Available at: https://www.frontiersin.org/journals/gastroenterology/articles/10.3389/fgstr.2022.987713/full.

Kim, M.S., Straesser, M.D., Keshavarz, B., et al. (2020) IgE to galactose-α-1,3-galactose wanes over time in patients who avoid tick bites. Journal of Allergy and Clinical Immunology: In Practice, 8(1), 364–367.e2. Available at: https://pmc.ncbi.nlm.nih.gov/articles/PMC6980488/.

Wilson, J.M., Keshavarz, B., Commins, S.P., et al. (2024) Tick bites, IgE to galactose-α-1,3-galactose and the alpha-gal syndrome. Allergy, 79(8), 1815–1828. Available at: https://onlinelibrary.wiley.com/doi/10.1111/all.16003.

Hawkins, R.B., Frisch, K., Dashiell, K., et al. (2020) Safety of intravenous heparin for cardiac surgery in patients with alpha-gal syndrome. The Annals of Thoracic Surgery, 110(3), 1035–1041. Available at: https://pmc.ncbi.nlm.nih.gov/articles/PMC8019687/.

Nwamara, U., Kilgore, K., Stirling, L. and El-Boghdadly, K. (2022) A retrospective evaluation of heparin product reactions in patients with alpha-gal allergy. Journal of Cardiothoracic and Vascular Anesthesia, 36(10), 3828–3833. Available at: https://pubmed.ncbi.nlm.nih.gov/34798527/.

Behmer, R.G., Thomas, R.S. and Goodine, R. (2022) Urticarial rash due to subcutaneous heparin in alpha-gal allergy. Journal of Maine Medical Center, 4(2), Article 9. Available at: https://knowledgeconnection.mainehealth.org/cgi/viewcontent.cgi?article=1122&context=jmmc.

Stone, C.A. Jr., Liu, Y., Relling, M.V., et al. (2017) Anaphylaxis after zoster vaccine: implicating alpha-gal. Journal of Allergy and Clinical Immunology: In Practice, 5(5), 1411–1413. Available at: https://pubmed.ncbi.nlm.nih.gov/27986511/.

Zafar, S., Ahmed, S.R., Nanda, A., et al. (2022) Are gelatin-containing vaccines safe to give in alpha-gal–sensitized patients?. Journal of Allergy and Clinical Immunology, 149(5), 1685–1687. Available at: https://www.jacionline.org/article/S0091-6749(21)02171-0/fulltext.

AAAAI (American Academy of Allergy, Asthma & Immunology) (2021) Alpha-gal syndrome and perioperative concerns (Ask the Expert). . Available at: https://www.aaaai.org/allergist-resources/ask-the-expert/answers/2021/periop.

Ailsworth, S.M., Hernandez, J., Patel, V., et al. (2024) Alpha-gal IgE prevalence patterns in the United States. Journal of Allergy and Clinical Immunology: In Practice, 12(5), —. Available at: https://www.jaci-inpractice.org/article/S2213-2198(23)01201-1/abstract.

www.ingramcontent.com/pod-product-compliance
Lightning Source LLC
Chambersburg PA
CBHW071428090426
42737CB00011B/1597